STRATEGIC SKILLS FOR PUBLIC HEALTH PRACTICE SERIES

Community Engagement

For access to digital chapters, visit the APHA Press bookstore (www.apha.org).

Strategic Skills for Public Health Practice Series
Series Editors: Michael Fraser, PhD, MS, and Brian C. Castrucci, DrPH

1. *Systems and Strategic Thinking*
2. *Policy Engagement*
3. *Resource Management and Finance*
4. *Community Engagement*
5. *Advancing Equity and Justice*
6. *Effective Communication*
7. *Change Management*
8. *Data-Based Decision Making*
9. *Cross-Sectoral Partnerships*

STRATEGIC SKILLS FOR PUBLIC HEALTH PRACTICE

SERIES

Community Engagement

Emily Yu, MBA
Editor

APHA PRESS
AN IMPRINT OF AMERICAN PUBLIC HEALTH ASSOCIATION

American Public Health Association
800 I Street, NW
Washington, DC 20001-3710
www.apha.org

Georges C. Benjamin, MD, MACP, Executive Director

Printed and bound in the United States of America
Book Production Editor: Maya Ribault
Typesetting: KnowledgeWorks Global, Ltd.
Cover Design: Alan Giarcanella
Printing and Binding: Sheridan Books

Library of Congress Cataloging-in-Publication Data

Names: Yu, Emily (Community health consultant), editor.
Title: Strategic skills : community engagement / edited by Emily Yu, MBA.
Description: Washington, DC : American Public Health Association, [2022] | Includes bibliographical references and index. | Summary: "Communities are dynamic and complex ecosystems that are constantly developing, changing, and evolving. The stories in this book bring forth an array of new ideas and questions for public health leaders about the important role and inherent power of communities in advancing better health for all"-- Provided by publisher.
Identifiers: LCCN 2022041947 (print) | LCCN 2022041948 (ebook) | ISBN 9780875533308 (paperback) | ISBN 9780875533315 (adobe pdf)
Subjects: LCSH: Community health services--United States. | Public health--United States. | Community organization--United States.
Classification: LCC RA445 .S75 2022 (print) | LCC RA445 (ebook) | DDC 362.10973--dc23/eng/20220928
LC record available at https://lccn.loc.gov/2022041947
LC ebook record available at https://lccn.loc.gov/2022041948

This book is dedicated to every person who believes in their community and is working to ensure a healthier tomorrow for all those who call it home.

Contents

Strategic Skills for Public Health Practice Series Introduction

Over the last 15 years, governmental public health professionals and partners nationwide have worked to define core competencies, essential services, and foundational capabilities of the public health.[1,2,3] Central to all these efforts is the public health workforce—the practitioners who work in local, state, territorial, tribal, and federal public health agencies to prevent disease and protect and promote the health of the public.

The governmental public health workforce is diverse and comprised of many technical specialties and professions. These professional identities have shaped public health practice and formed categories of work that comprise the organizational chart most governmental public health agencies utilize, such as maternal and child health, environmental health, epidemiology and surveillance, communicable disease control, administration and finance, school health, and several others.

These categories have served public health well by helping organize work and allowing for professionalization and leadership development within specific areas. Over 21 national professional associations represent categorical or function areas within state and territorial health departments alone, not to mention peer groups and affinity groups that are part of the Association of State and Territorial Health Officials and other allied organizations such as the National Association of County and City Health Officials, the Big Cities Health Coalition, CityMatCH (urban maternal and child health programs), the National Environmental Health Association, and others.

These specialty designations have also led to fragmentation within agencies at a time when government is attempting to align more nimbly to meet the needs of the jurisdictions they serve. Few public health professionals have formal training in the skills needed to successfully adapt their work to navigate these changes, especially the strategic skills needed to position their work to meet contemporary public health challenges that require inter- and intra-agency collaboration for success. For example, the pressures and challenges imposed on the public health ecosystem and its workers by the COVID-19 pandemic illustrate the urgency of preparing the public health workforce not just for technical challenges but also for strategic and adaptive challenges posed by novel health threats that require an "all of government" approach to resolve.

Several external forces in recent years, including the movement from Public Health 2.0 to Public Health 3.0 and the six-year-long, three-phased Public Health Workforce Interests and Needs Survey, have either advocated for or implied the need for complementing the workforce's existing discipline-specific expertise with developing a set of strategic skills.

In 2017, the de Beaumont Foundation spearheaded the development of the National Consortium for Public Health Workforce Development comprised of public health leaders from 34 national partner organizations representing a variety of disciplines and settings nationwide. The Consortium was established "to communicate the needs of the front-line public health worker to national partners and funders."[4]

By consensus, the Consortium identified the following nine "indispensable, high-performance skills applicable to the entire public health workforce regardless of specialty or discipline."[5]

- Systems and strategic thinking
- Change management
- Effective communication
- Data-driven decision making
- Community engagement
- Justice, equity, diversity, and inclusion
- Resource management and finance
- Policy engagement
- Cross-sectoral partnerships

These strategic skills are needed by specialty-specific, technical experts in order to realize the multisector, cross-cutting visionary leadership needed today. The Consortium's "call to action" paper asserted this challenge to public health educators: "While maintaining excellence in core scientific disciplines continues to be a priority, developers and deliverers of public health education and training need to act in new and different ways if the governmental public health workforce is to gain competency in the strategic skills needed throughout the entire public health workforce."[5]

Creating these "new and different ways" of building public health workforce competencies in the strategic skills should be a priority for academic programs, professional associations, and public health partners nationwide. This Strategic Skills Series presents a new way to expand the education and training of the public health workforce, equipping its members for multisector collaboration to create policies and programs intended to solve real problems.

To develop this series, we have recruited thought leaders and experts to serve as the authors of each volume. The consistent format applied to each book in the series is intended to facilitate the learner's absorption and retention of key concepts and applications. The practice-based objectives of each book in the series are described below:

- **Systems and strategic thinking:** Grasp patterns and relationships to understand systems contributing to public health problems and identify high-impact interventions.
- **Change management:** Scale programs in response to the changing environments and shape core elements that sustain programs in challenge and crisis.
- **Effective communication:** Convey resonant, compelling public health messages to broad audiences—the public, partners, and policymakers.
- **Data-driven decision making:** Leverage, synthesize, and analyze multiple sources of electronic data and use informatics to identify and act on health priorities, population impacts, evidence-based approaches, and health and cost-related outcomes.
- **Community engagement:** Describe the most effective methods of and the beneficial outcomes from engaging communities in promoting health and well-being. Promote the model of equitable distribution of decision-making power.
- **Justice, equity, diversity, and inclusion:** Understand and respond to the changing demographics of the US population and the public health workforce itself. Seek out, listen to, include, and promote underrepresented populations in reaching effective health solutions.
- **Resource management and finance:** Oversee recruitment, acquisition, and retention of the workforce and manage fiscal resources responsibly.
- **Policy engagement:** Address public health concerns and needs and engage effectively with local, state, and federal policymakers and partners.
- **Cross-sectoral partnerships:** Bring together two or more distinct fields (e.g., health care and transportation) for greater impact so that public health professionals can maintain long-term collaborations that combine a unique set of resources, experience, and knowledge to effectively address multifaceted issues (e.g., the social determinants of health).

As we aim to move public health forward to meet the challenges of contemporary practice, we are excited to edit each of these volumes. It is our fervent hope that each of the books in this series represents a significant brick in the foundation of developing your capacity to address today's urgencies as well as tomorrow's opportunities and challenges.

Michael Fraser, PhD, MS
Brian C. Castrucci, DrPH

REFERENCES

1. Public Health Foundation. Core competencies for public health professionals. 2014. Available at: http://www.phf.org/programs/corecompetencies/Pages/Core_Competencies_Domains.aspx. Accessed January 22, 2021.
2. US Centers for Disease Control and Prevention. 10 essential public health services. 2020. Available at: https://www.cdc.gov/publichealthgateway/publichealthservices/essentialhealthservices.html. Accessed January 22, 2021.

3. Public Health National Center for Innovation. Foundational public health services. 2018. Available at: https://phnci.org/uploads/resource-files/FPHS-Factsheet-November-2018.pdf. Accessed January 22, 2021.
4. de Beaumont Foundation. Building skills for a more strategic public health workforce: a call to action. 2019. Available at: https://debeaumont.org/wp-content/uploads/2019/04/Building-Skills-for-a-More-Strategic-Public-Health-Workforce.pdf. Accessed September 26, 2022.
5. de Beaumont Foundation. Building skills for a more strategic public health workforce: a call to action. July 18, 2017. Available at: https://www.debeaumont.org/news/2017/building-skills-for-a-more-strategic-health-workforce-a-call-to-action. Accessed January 22, 2021.

Preface

Communities are dynamic and complex ecosystems that are constantly developing, changing, and evolving. Made up of different individuals, organizations, and infrastructure, each one is rich with its own identity, culture, and history. And while every community may be unique, the people within them all have one thing in common—they want to thrive, whether that be socially, economically, and/or culturally.

As public health practitioners, we are able to support community members and help them realize this goal through the lens of health equity. Doing so requires us to center community members in our efforts to ensure that everyone has the opportunity to be healthy and thrive. Achieving such an important and urgent objective requires us to reimagine how we define, operationalize, and evaluate community engagement. By focusing on the building of power, capacity, and relationships among residents and those most affected by the issues being considered, our efforts have the potential to drive sustainable improvements in health within a community.

For many of us working in the field of community health, the reality we must contend with is that the systems currently in place—in our organizations and communities—often limit or work against our efforts to engage with, and center, community. Take for example deficit-based framing, resident disenfranchisement, short-term grant cycles, or disinvestment in local businesses and organizations. Changing these norms and practices requires us to reflect on our role within the community, the power we and our organizations possess, and the requisite shift in mindset of what engagement with community means, looks like, and feels like.

In developing this book, I asked each contributor to complete this very task—to not only reflect on but also to define what community engagement means to them. Upon my reading the submissions, several key themes presented themselves: alignment, balance of power, and collaboration. When considered in concert, these three themes, or the ABCs, serve as helpful concepts while reading this book and ultimately considering not only what community engagement is but also how to center it.

THEME 1: ALIGNMENT

Community engagement is defined by inclusive community-centered decision-making. Good community engagement happens when residents, workforce, governments, and organizations work together transparently to create and bring into being sustainable solutions for their community's present and future. It's about listening to and supporting communities to build long-term relationships and develop meaningful solutions to complex issues.

Evette De Luca
The Social Impact Artists

Community engagement is building genuine, inclusive, and diverse relationships. It is a continuous exchange and sharing of ideas, information, and resources to understand the experience, needs, and priorities of a community. It allows the community to lead the work and share in decision-making regarding changes to policies, programs, services, and practices.

Sarah Garber, MS
Missoula City-County Health Department

Community engagement is actively listening with an open heart and mindset by accepting the community members as they are; being transparent with your purpose; leaving behind all implicit and explicit bias, stereotypes; and seeing residents as individuals who love their communities.

Natasha Butler, CHW, CHWI
Maternal Upstream Management

THEME 2: BALANCE OF POWER

To me, community engagement, really, is the shift of power from institutions to communities. When we are truly and actively engaged with our community, we begin to move our institutions to be about service instead of authority and control. And when we lead with love for our communities, we build true partnerships that will achieve our shared goals.

Jennifer Muggeo, MPH
Ledge Light Health District

To build power with community residents that transforms resources, budgets and policies into a gift for an equitable, joyful, and healthy community for all.

Lisa Beczkiewicz
Missoula City-County Health Department

Community engagement means to center residents in initiatives that will impact them. Centering residents builds power and capacity in the community, strengthening their ability to hold institutions accountable, to be responsive to their community goals and leverage their collective assets, to create a future of their own design that meets their priorities and takes into account their lived experience as expertise.

Melissa Monbouquette, MPA
The BUILD Health Challenge

1. We need to intentionally have community at the table from the onset and throughout. We must ensure that the community voice is heard, valued, and respected.
2. We must create a new balance of power. We do it by ensuring that every individual, family, and community has a voice.
3. We must ask "What is needed?" before we act and not assume we know what is best for the communities and the individuals we serve.

Ana P. Novais
Rhode Island Executive Office of Health
and Human Services

Community engagement is a strategic process and commitment to center the experience and desires of the people in a community (geographic or otherwise) in creating positive change.

Jessica Mulcahy, MA
Success Measures at NeighborWorks America

THEME 3: COLLABORATION

Community engagement is the process and outcome of creating relationships with community to achieve long-term and sustainable change. It is a conscious decision to be collaborative to improve the health of a community.

James Bell III, DSW
Just Solutions LLC

It is a process of working together with a particular group of people (defined by geography, race, ethnicity, socioeconomic status, etc.) to address issues that affect the well-being and quality of life of said community.

Manuel J. Castañeda, MS, MJ
New Brunswick Tomorrow

Community engagement is about building authentic relationships, respecting and connecting with leaders in the community to deepen the work and trust of the community.

Community engagement is a long-term proposition and reiterative because goals, needs, and vision can shift over time; adjustment is a natural part of the process.

Kim Foreman
Environmental Health Watch

The intentional incorporation of community voices and concerns into existing public health strategies and civic programs in a manner that includes community members at all stages. Maintaining the involvement of the community from problem identification through implementation and assessment of outcomes is central to true community engagement.

Patrick J. Cusick, MSPH, REHS
Cleveland Department of Public Health

Community engagement is the development of relationships, including communication and maintenance of those relationships; the building of resources and providing access for those being engaged; and the solid codevelopment of processes that both inspire people and reciprocally create impact toward the purpose of the engagement.

C. Benzel Jimmerson
Metro DEEP, Metropolitan Diversity
and Economic Equity Partners

Connections that go deeper, that facilitate trust and bind us in shared experience. Community engagement has to mean integration above participation. Communities and families know their needs best. Holding space for our connected stories helps us to listen for understanding and lasting systemic change. Together we rise!

Nichelle Gilbert
Partnership for Community Action

While there is no one definition or universal playbook when it comes to community engagement, a fundamental step for those looking to engage more effectively with community is understanding what it is and why it matters. This book endeavors to support practitioners by bringing to life concepts related to the ABCs through the insights, experiences, and perspectives shared therein. Chapter 1 begins by spotlighting community voices and their perspectives on what it means to work with and for the community. Chapter 2 provides readers with insights into what a community is and how stakeholders, specifically residents and organizations, can align for greater impact. Next, Chapters 3 and 4 introduce and unpack various frames supporting the concept and act of community engagement. Finally, the book ends with a collection of brief and diverse examples of community engagement from across the country that exemplify many of the concepts and ideas shared in earlier chapters.

Before you dive into this book, I invite you to consider what your own definition of community engagement is and to pause again after you've read the book to take note of how, if at all, it has changed. My hope is that these stories will inspire an array of new ideas and questions for public health leaders about the important role and inherent power of communities in advancing better health for all.

Emily Yu, MBA

1

Letters to the Field of Public Health: Community Leaders Define What Community Engagement Means to Them

Melissa Monbouquette, MPA, Manuel J. Castañeda, MS, MJ, Nichelle Gilbert, Natasha Butler, CHW, CHWI, and C. Benzel Jimmerson

INTRODUCTION: CENTERING LIVED EXPERIENCE AS EXPERTISE IN COMMUNITY ENGAGEMENT

Melissa Monbouquette, MPA

Definitions of community engagement can have different meanings for different people. Depending on the community, sector, and history of the relationship, those processes may fall anywhere along the spectrum of public participation put forth by the International Association for Public Participation: informing, consulting, involving, collaborating, or empowering.[1] However, it is in the latter two—accountable collaboration and power building—that we see meaningful change by allowing the experience and vision of those impacted to be the driver of the path forward. To ensure that community members are centered in the work, organizations must reduce barriers to participation in decision-making processes, ensure that strategies are aligned with community priorities, and create a culture of accountability, healing, and trust.

When embarking on a community engagement process, we must be mindful that sometimes the priorities of a community may not be the same as the priorities of the institutions, policymakers, administrators, and others who serve them. Even when the overall target issue is aligned, the desired approach may be different. For example, while a community development agency may be advocating for a long-term policy change to preserve affordable housing, residents in that neighborhood might be concerned about where they will sleep at the end of the week. This is not to say that residents don't want long-term changes—of course they do—but the first step must be to ensure that any physiological human needs are met and in a way that is culturally appropriate. Proposed solutions are often packaged by social-change makers in the form of a program, but they can only be as effective as residents have time, resources, and interest in participating in them. Moreover, asking residents to contribute to an initiative without making sure that it is what they want and that they are safe, healthy, and resourced may ultimately result in an exploitive exchange and serve only to exacerbate distrust.

Acknowledging and reducing barriers to access and participation can be challenging for public health practitioners. Reducing barriers may carry an unexpected financial weight or feel like a distraction from the long-term goal, but in truth doing this cannot be an either/or question. Human need must be addressed now and until no longer necessary; at the same time, we cannot as a society—and as fellow humans—watch these needs perpetuate without planning for sustainable, systemic changes that can reduce them. By addressing critical need first, we create an opportunity for meaningful connections and building a relationship.

Beyond that, residents have a right to work on their own self-identified long-term goals and to say no to well-meaning but misdirected attempts to push them in a different direction. Developer and activist Majora Carter shares the example of a local councilman who threatened to veto any housing development in the South Bronx that wasn't 100% affordable, whereas she and others who live there preferred mixed-income housing that would incentivize residents who have the means for economic investment to stay in the neighborhood, prevent brain drain, and reduce concentrated poverty.[2] Demonstrating that we understand each other's priorities and will support each other in achieving them develops trust, which is in turn foundational for authentic partnership and sustained impact moving forward.

Listening to community voice is the first step, as residents carry systemic injustices with them and are best equipped to articulate the impact. That expertise and those connections should be recognized as central to the success of our collaborative efforts and compensated as such. This is particularly important, as the vision and ability to execute the vision are often already there, despite being undervalued and hamstrung by systemic barriers. Rethinking and resourcing this work is critical.

It is also important to acknowledge that many large institutions have been complicit participants in a white supremacist, patriarchal, and ableist culture; this is not surprising, considering the long and ongoing history of embedded discrimination in the United States. Residents often have stories of how powerful institutions have created or perpetuated harm in communities of color, including bias in access to services (or refusal of services); policies that exacerbate inequity; displacement; and discriminatory hiring practices. In Greensboro, North Carolina, when a hospital representative pointed to segregated medical policies that lasted into the 1960s and the decades it took to acknowledge and

> Lived experience is expertise. No one knows better what a culturally inclusive intervention looks like than members of the culture. No one can bring along other residents and neighbors more than those who live in the neighborhood. No one is more capable of assessing the impact of an issue than those who have lived through it, and no one has a clearer vision of what solutions would effect meaningful change than those who would experience it.

apologize for these practices as an example of a lingering wound, a community partner said that the "unprompted statement inspired her to do even more to bring residents to the table with the health system to work together" toward a better future.[3] By acknowledging that history and participating in dialogue with community members where they are located, institutions can begin to create space for honesty and accountability—and for the first steps toward repair, healing, and thriving.

Centering residents in this work builds power and resources in the community; it fosters the ability to hold institutions accountable, to be responsive to their community goals and leverage their collective assets, and to create a future of their own design that meets their priorities and takes into account their lived expertise. Building civic, political, and economic power for those who are historically shut out of the process is transformative and can activate entire communities. This is justice, not only utilizing an equity lens to reduce health disparities but also focusing on changing systems to create a "shared affirmative vision of a fair and inclusive society."[4] To do so, we must work to realign power and resources around the community.

So, if this understanding of the past and what is needed now helps pave a path forward to center community, what is the role for government agencies, funders, health care systems, and others? If a rebalancing of power is needed, how can and should these institutions find new ways to support communities—in particular, communities in search of health equity and racial justice? We must come together in the cocreation of a new, aligned model for health that addresses upstream health disparities at their root. Resident voices are at the heart of this vision.

The truth is that no one will get community partnership right perfectly the first time, or sometimes even after many attempts down the road. Even with the best of intentions, there will be systemic barriers to overcome, unlearning to be done, and unintended hurt to address. There will be tough conversations and tough decisions. But as you will see in the three "letters from the field" in this chapter, while the work is slow and challenging, it is also deeply energizing and impactful. We know what the best practices are, and if we listen, we continue to learn as we go. Our best chance of improving health for all is to make sure that those who are most affected by unjust systems are the voices centered in the decision-making, planning, and implementation processes—and in so doing, we hold ourselves accountable to change these systems accordingly.

COMMUNITY LEADERS FOSTER COMMUNITY ENGAGEMENT

Manuel J. Castañeda, MS, MJ

My name is Manuel Castañeda and I have lived in New Brunswick, New Jersey, for most of my life. New Brunswick is much more than the place where I live and work, it's home. Professionally, I've dedicated myself to community service, starting out by advocating and providing services for people living with HIV/AIDS to my current position as director of community health at New Brunswick Tomorrow (NBT; for more on the organization, see: https://www.nbtomorrow.org). A social impact organization, NBT is dedicated to enriching the lives of New Brunswick residents by fostering public and private networks of institutions and community organizations and serving as a catalyst in developing and supporting solutions that improve the quality of life in our community. The organization has focused on addressing the issues that matter most to city residents and families. We believe that the true revitalization of any city must put people at the center of its activities.

Community engagement has been defined with its fair share of variations, but at its core, I have come to see that it involves a process of working together with a particular group of people (e.g., defined by geography, race, ethnicity, socioeconomic status) to address issues that affect the well-being and, particularly in my case, health outcomes of said community.

The variations within definition and practice depend on the level of community engagement applied. In order to be effective, community engagement needs to move beyond community *participation* to community *integration,* from *identifying* the prevalent community issues to *developing, implementing, and evaluating* strategic plans to address issues. We as community health leaders need to move beyond working *for* the community and move toward working *with* the community as an equal strategic partner. This is where I believe we as practitioners need to improve if we are ever to really have a positive impact within the communities we're working with.

Community engagement begins with community members helping in identifying the community issue to be addressed and playing an active role in the development of the solution. As practitioners, we have to avoid being prescriptive and assuming that the issue we see as most relevant is that which is worth addressing. The truth is, both stakeholders in the community have an important role to play—together. A synergy or agreement on the issue in question is needed between practitioners and community members in order to truly achieve community buy-in.

A key lesson learned is that identifying, developing (if needed), and employing community leaders is essential for effective community engagement. Therefore, ensuring that community members are part of the initiative from its development through implementation is key. A prime example is our community health ambassadors (CHAs), who are an integral part of our New Brunswick Healthy Housing Collaborative. They are New Brunswick residents who have decided to do their part to better their community and who recognize the importance of promoting health and wellness (see Figure 1-1, Community Health Workers). For a city that has a substantial marginalized population (i.e., racial minorities, undocumented residents, and low-income families), there is a lot of distrust of those outside the community irrespective of their intentions. Our CHAs help better engage the community by serving as the cultural bridge between community-based organizations, health care agencies, and their respective communities.

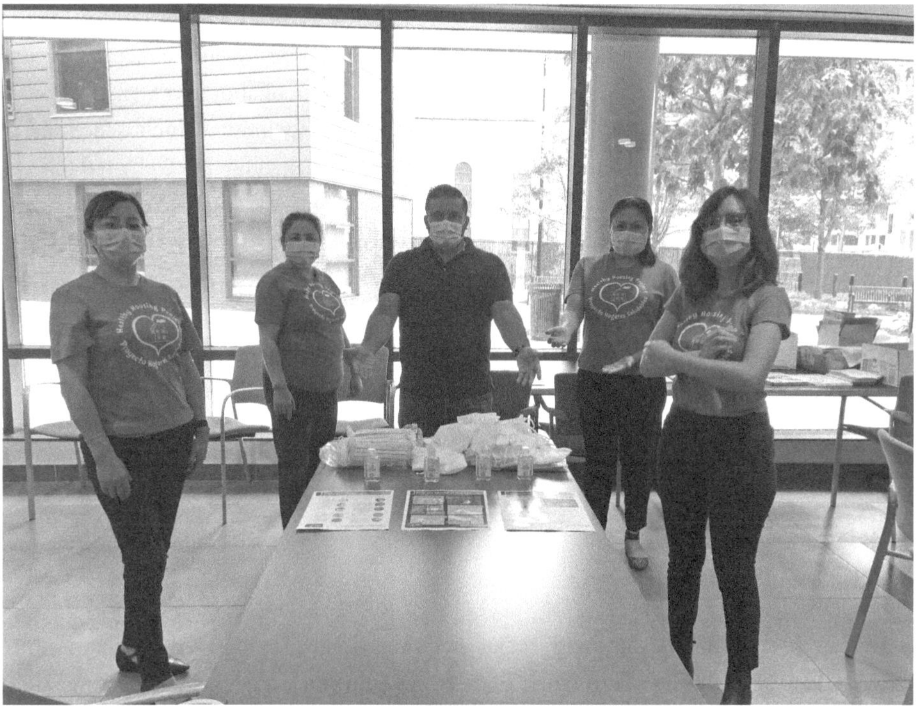

Source: Reprinted with permission of New Brunswick Tomorrow.

Figure 1-1. Community Health Workers

Not only do CHAs serve as the bridge to get "in the door" but their peer-to-peer interaction is also an effective approach to ensure that residents receive and have access to information about our focused health initiatives and how these are designed to support them and the community. In other words, they help ensure that the message is not only understood but also relevant and accepted. They also provide necessary feedback that gives valuable community insight and critique of the initiative to help ensure that our project is internally and externally relevant to the community. Their contributions to the project propelled our efforts overall. For example, we had only about 12 home assessments scheduled within the community in the early stages of our healthy housing initiative. In contrast, the CHAs were able to get over 90 residents signed up for home assessments within one community event, leading to over 200 homes being assessed to date and helping us surpass our target goal, providing us the data necessary to identify the prevalent housing issues facing New Brunswick residents.

With respect to having community members involved in the development and implementation of initiatives to address our healthy housing issues, the institutional partners worked closely with the CHAs to design a two-part approach. The first part included providing CHAs with the tools and training to become tenant rights advocates.

Known as the "ladies in the red shirts," they have become a community resource in their own right and proactively engage with residents on housing and health concerns. As an established community resource, the Healthy Housing Collaborative's institutional partners then worked with the CHAs to develop a tenant association, which is facilitated by the CHAs to address community housing concerns. It is through the CHA-led tenant association that we are currently in the process of working with the City of New Brunswick to enact a city ordinance that will address water utility charges to ensure tenants are paying only their fair share of the water bill.

All in all, CHA contributions provide a unique service for community members to overcome system barriers, learn about the importance of healthy housing and tenant rights, and become community advocates that affect policy change as a means to truly help create a culture of healthy housing in our community.

TOGETHER WE RISE

Nichelle Gilbert

Every day we stand face to face with racial inequities that are embedded deeply into the systems that shape our lives, our work, and our communities. Systems-level change that supports strong, healthy communities where everyone has the opportunity to thrive requires our collective investment in people, a connection to leadership and agency, and community-led solutions. It requires community engagement. The act of community engagement and building of community power is rooted in deeply personal relationships. These connections require time, trust, and an acknowledgment and reverence for lived experience.

Inclusivity in decision-making is at the core of this work. Engagement requires community-driven strategies to create race-conscious, equitable practices. Popular education strategies shape the work we do alongside the community, acknowledging and respecting the expertise brought by all. Everyone is a teacher, and we are all learners. Program development and strategic direction solicit community participation and true integration, and we believe that together we rise. It is with this grounding that the Partnership for Community Action (PCA) was created to help build relational power, create enduring relationships, develop collective leadership, design innovative solutions, and advocate for a stronger New Mexico (for more on PCA, see: https://www.forcommunityaction.org).

Through the application of traditional community-organizing strategies, PCA has worked to build strong, healthy communities in Albuquerque's South Valley and across New Mexico since 1990. Our organization focuses on critical community issues, including education, economic sustainability, health equity, and immigrant rights. Through raising awareness and advocacy opportunities, we support people and families to become

> By embracing these community-centered values, we work on behalf of no one, but alongside change agents and disruptors of inequitable and oppressive systems as equals.

strong leaders in their neighborhoods and in New Mexico. We envision strong, healthy communities in which everyone has access to quality education, wellness, and economic opportunity, starting locally and spreading across New Mexico.

Our impact is driven by the fundamental understanding that our neighbors are the drivers and the foundation of their communities. We know that when everyday people and their families prosper, we all succeed. Over the last 30 years, we at PCA have learned that to achieve meaningful systems change, to support community health, and to develop strong community leaders and advocates, we as intermediaries, community-based organizations, and community health champions must take a number of important steps:

- Help to support community to take ownership of solutions and lead the way;
- Invest in people and work in deeply personal ways alongside community to engage them in public life to take action around the issues that most affect their lives;
- Help to develop strong leaders who are effective advocates for their families and their communities through education, training, and a commitment to enduring relationships;
- Organize communities by encouraging families, neighborhoods, and institutions to come together around issues they care about and thereby advance community-led solutions; and
- Advocate for systemic change that improves opportunity for all.

As a grassroots organizing nonprofit, we early on made the decision that our work would center on community voice. It is clear that everyday community leaders are the true experts when it comes to knowing what they and their families need to thrive. Still, families and the voices of community members all too often go unheard in the conversations that affect them the most. Understanding that people know their own communities best, we support families in taking ownership of the solutions and lead the way. By connecting communities to decision makers, we can create lasting change together.

THE UNTOLD, REAL STORY OF ALIEF

Natasha Butler, CHW, CHWI

Alief is a suburb of Houston, Texas. The community is a little over 100 years old and was founded as a rural farm town. When it was founded, it was an all-white community until the late 1970s. In the early 1980s, African Americans started moving in from areas inside the loop to find better schools and newer housing options. The diversity of the community increased with Hispanic and Asian populations as well, and Alief became an incredibly diverse community. However, it was not always this way.

During the 1990s, affluent white residents moved out of Alief to wealthier communities such as Katy and River Oaks. In 1985, Alief was annexed to become part of the City of Houston. Shortly thereafter, the first library opened, and West Houston Medical Center was built. In the late 1990s, the population demographics changed again. Over 70 languages were spoken and white flight was increasing, truly becoming a real experience. Despite minority populations being the largest demographics, remaining white residents continued to retain leadership roles within local systems, including education, health care, and community groups such as Alief Super Neighborhood Council, International Management District, and Westchase Management District. Even now, in 2022, the leadership of Alief still looks the same as it did decades ago, despite the more than 100 languages now being spoken by a very diverse community.

Underlying these challenges are significant disparities, among them high rates of poverty and infant and maternal morbidity, as well as the lack of access to healthy food and health care. It is because of these social determinants of health that our work with The BUILD Health Challenge (BUILD), a national awards program designed to advance health equity by strengthening cross-sector collaboratives and implementing community-driven approaches, has been transformative. It has been not just about collecting data but also about changing mindsets. It has allowed us to elevate the voices of those impacted by bringing others to the table. We have realized that we needed to create community-based organizations to address these issues through advocacy, empowerment, and removal of barriers that have been allowing our community to experience decline over the years. People of color are now speaking up and having tough, critical conversations with white people about systemic racism in our community and how to do transformative work.

Our "Letters to the Field of Public Health," starting with mine, seek to elevate the young people of Alief, whose voices have been ignored and who are now advocating for systemic change via community engagement. To protect the privacy of the teens, their names are not included at their request.

Natasha's Story

As a community advocate with over 20 years of experience, I thought I had a great knowledge of effective community engagement. While attending college, I completed training in a leadership group that focused on best practices to engage communities. The training was taught by a professor who was an effective lobbyist for Planned Parenthood. Her words of wisdom and experiences seemed as if they would work on every community. She explained that leaders should use best practices to engage with community using a traditional model of hosting meetings, forming focus groups, finding experts with community development degrees, and working with city planning departments to build communities.

Well, these skills worked for a little while in my life until I moved into my community home. I found that my community is not a traditional community, as there are over 100 languages spoken. None of the academic skills I learned in college were effective. I had to reconcile to the reality that equity was going to be needed to address real issues affecting my community, so I had to create a grassroots level of community engagement. I learned that I needed to make sure that those who were directly affected needed to be providing their input and needed to be in leadership spaces to advocate effectively for themselves. In 2021, I became part of the BUILD 3.0 cohort, and I experienced another mindset change regarding community engagement. Our BUILD project has a special population of teen mothers. These young moms have taught me great lessons in the field that I want to share with anyone trying to do real community engagement.

Teen 1's Story

People talk about my community apathy. They have a term called "Alief Apathy." This refers to the way that our community does not get involved in projects, voting, community meetings, forums, or community volunteer events. Well, it is not Alief apathy that explains the lack of involvement in community. It is not that I do not care. It is that maybe I do not care about what others care about. In my community, there is a community group that focuses on pets, trees, and crime. These things don't matter to me, but I do care about my community. I just care about other things such as health care, schools, jobs, parks, and libraries. Also, I just have more important things in my life that don't allow me to attend all these community spaces. I work two jobs, attend school, and take care of my siblings. I just don't have a lot of extra time to give away for projects that don't matter to me. I would rather focus my time on things and people that are important to me. I do care, just not about the things that a small group of 70-year-old white women care about who are the representatives for our community.

> How about asking me what I do care about and adding that into the projects. My voice matters and it deserves to be heard. Invite me to the table, actively listen to me, and see me even in my youth that I have value.

Teen 2's Story

When I was a child, my mom and abuela taught me not to open the door for strangers, not to talk to strangers, and not to give our information to strangers. Every week, there is some new group trying to engage the community by knocking on doors and

> That is why we do not open the door. We do not know you. You do not live in our neighborhood, you do not look like us in racial diversity, and you talk to us as if we do not know our own community.

asking me to share personal information. If police, parents, and adults are telling the community not to open doors to strangers, why are people trying to use this method to engage our community? Last year, people from the census were knocking on doors the same time as criminals were impersonating police officers to gain access to people's homes. This goes against all the safety procedures in my house and the houses of most people in our community.

The other issue is that people keep wanting us to fill out surveys and asking personal questions. Would you give personal information to a stranger? Would you want to spend 15 minutes answering questions from a stranger, but when you ask them what they are doing with the responses, they say they are just collecting data for some project. There's never real follow-up with the group; they don't leave any contact information or even allow you to look up the project. So, I say to people who are door knocking and taking surveys in my community, people are not allowed to wander around in your gated neighborhoods and go door to door, so please stop doing it in my neighborhood.

Teen 3's Story

Why is it that people come into my community when they're working on some special project, trying to get money, or want me to sign up for someone's campaign? My community is missing resources like parks, healthy grocery stores, clinics, libraries, jobs, clean drinking water, sidewalks, streetlights, and safe neighborhoods. The only time I see people from the outside, elected officials, block walkers, and lobbyist groups, it is for me to engage in your projects, take a photo with you, sign some petition, or sign up to help you with some project. My community is not here to be used for your selfish purpose because we are a poor community. We don't want you to be our voice for your purpose. If you are not willing to roll up your sleeves, donate money, or provide resources to our community, stop wasting both of our time.

> We do not want to be used for political campaigns, photo shoots, or to get your numbers that you need for your service project. We deserve better and that is why we keep telling you "No thank you," "We are not interested," or "I do not have time." Our community engagement is about activism in our community for our community.

Teen 4's Story

People are always talking about how we as young people use technology to bully people, find friends, date, bank, and such. It is because we are a generation that has had technology in every part of our lives. Technology is an easy way to communicate to a large group. You can get 100 people on a zoom call, but it is a lot harder to get 100 people to come to a community meeting. Do we have to all be in the same place to be effective? Community engagement is using the tools that are available to engage all people. We're stuck in this thought process of we have always done things this way. My community is a very young community, but our leaders are 70 years old and don't see the value in using technology to engage us. They want us to use their traditional ways. They have meetings during the day while most people in the community are either working or in school. It makes a person wonder if you have meetings during the times when you know we are busy, is that an intentional way to limit our voices. We're taking back our voices by hosting our own meetings when we're available and using the tools we prefer. So, we as young people are rising up and activating in the best way we know how, and that is using technology.

> Yes, we have had to start our own organization, but when you cannot change a person's mindset, be the change you seek.

THE POWER OF HUMAN CONNECTION

C. Benzel Jimmerson

Have you ever heard the adage "Understanding is to the heart what air is to the body" or "People will not remember what you say as much as how you made them feel"? This is truth. In fact, these truths are at the core of two of the most highly missed and underrated elements when it comes to the best practices of community engagement: the ability to connect in the first place and ensuring authentic relationships are the only necessary result. Everything else will follow.

It takes a very special person to be able to connect, especially when doing so across cultural, economic, and experiential lines. To understand this significance, think about famous psychologists or therapists such as Sigmund Freud or Alfred Alder. Some just had innate abilities that not only allowed them to produce phenomenal results with whomever they worked with but also led to the creation of modalities that have now been taught to students for generations.

In this information age, multitudes of people are developing their own modalities, curriculum, and methods of connection. Only a select, special few can effectively connect to others. And not just with their natural circle but with the masses. Certainly, more people now have access to others and the opportunity to make connections, but doing so is still the exception. So, if you are trying to connect with a community you are not from, it is imperative that you either have that special gift of connection or find people who do, people who are already trusted by and integrated with the community you hope to connect with.

The pathway to the latter is via an ethnographic community development formula I created based on experiencing success using this and simple math. Use the base of 1 connector and then 10 × 10 = 100. Observing, interacting with, and genuinely connecting with people inside a targeted community or group, your goal is to establish an authentic relationship with at least one person who is an influencer. This influencer can either run point or lead you to another nine connectors. Those 10 connectors can then each repeat that model, being responsible for engaging 10 people apiece—a sustainable and duplicatable model: 10 engage 10.

Now we are back to 10 × 10 = 100. This concept I learned from two very important elders in my life, Ray Washington and Richard Male, both of whom have organized movements that resulted in global impacts. The foundations for meaningful engagement, or a movement, is solidified at 100 people. Does engaging 100 people feel daunting? It is for most of us. But 10, 10 is an extremely doable number of people to engage. So, 10 who each get 10 = 100. Authentic relationships combined with leveraging those connections within a duplicatable model ensure sustainable and deep community engagement.

Let us deepen the concept, starting with how one organization, Metro Diversity & Economic Equity Partners (DEEP), has in three short years gained the trust of a community (for more on Metro DEEP, see: https://www.metrodeep.com). This organization's approach has transformed paradigms, moving from a rocky starting place to wild success by building an ecosystem and infrastructure with enough results to resonate into a national expansion slated to take place by 2025.

Metro DEEP was built to connect, uplift, build out, and strategically integrate a Black economic ecosystem. Metro DEEP begins by learning about the people and culture in the area, listening deeply. It identifies both strengths and gaps, then connects with trusted, experienced, and influential leaders in the region, giving them ownership in the ensuing process to address an issue identified by the community. Then, the process of filling gaps by building up assets occurs.

We believe that collaboration, in and of itself, doesn't have real teeth. Rather, collaboration is a means to achieve an outcome. The achievement of alignment, or congruence, between stakeholders is what ultimately builds sustainable community engagement and real partnership. Consider a committed relationship or friendship. There must be an alignment of values, behaviors, and purpose; otherwise, it is temporary. To fill a temporary need is not bad in itself. Yet, it takes congruence and reciprocal commitment to each other, or the group, in order to form a lasting partnership. Often, a budget within a partnership is what seals the relationship.

We all have to find our niche and become the best at it until we are able to offer it as an expertise to other groups who are great at some other "lane." At this point in an organized movement, we can accelerate and begin lifting up those who do not have the access, the future orientation, the hope—those who lack the experience and expertise necessary to do more than survive. Now we have touched people in the ways they most need, affected their lives . . . this proves we have listened to their hearts, and they feel supported and therefore connected.

The pathway to strengthening community engagement can be summarized by the following seven elements—or as we call them at Metro DEEP, community integration marketing (CIM). When taken as a whole, practicing these seven areas can help support the sustainability of an organization and anchor it and its stakeholders within a particular community. The CIM approach is built to support the sustainability and anchoring of an organization, an institution, or simply a project within a particular community.*

1. Listen: Listening deeply and for clarity of what the people in the target group or community want and say they need. This must not be listening according to what *you* hope to accomplish, grant requirements, or any other bias.
2. Identify strengths and gaps: What people need is beyond what they already have. Therefore, by understanding the assets, you can see gaps without that being the focus.
3. Connect with trusted leaders and experts: Depending on your relationship to a community and the dynamics inside that community, connecting with trusted leaders and experts helps you be more open to, and understand, the views of the community. This direct connection is often a critical one because as an outsider you might not be told the truth or hear the whole truth.
4. Build congruence/partnerships: This is the hardest step. If not done right, true congruence cannot be achieved and can result in exploitive, harmful, or inauthentic partnerships. Ultimately, one to five real partnerships, depending on the scope of the project, may be all you need.
5. Build pipelines and culture: Once you have the foundations necessary to know you have integrated into a community, it is all about building new pathways. Figure out how to give power, economics, and leadership back to the community you are in.
6. Use automation: What allows you to step away or sleep while the work continues?
7. Enable legacy building (exit planning): The most successful things live on beyond our presence. Enable this legacy by planning today's purpose and impact while grooming tomorrow's leaders.

My final advice: be yourself no matter what, lead with genuine curiosity, and understand respect—not just "in your custom" or "being careful not to offend," but respect

*For a more detailed description of community integration marketing, visit the resources section of the Metro DEEP website at: www.metrodeep.com.

from human to human. Doing these three things *just as you are* will get you connected and keep you engaged just about anywhere in the world because people will sense your authenticity, and that is infectious in every language.

REFERENCES

1. International Association for Public Participation. IAP2 Spectrum of public participation. Available at: https://cdn.ymaws.com/www.iap2.org/resource/resmgr/pillars/Spectrum_8.5x11_Print.pdf. Accessed August 29, 2022.
2. Carter M. *Reclaiming Your Community: You Don't Have to Move Out of Your Neighborhood to Live in a Better One.* 1st ed. Oakland, CA: Berrett-Koehler; 2022:24.
3. Marple K. How a health system acknowledged historic racism to BUILD community trust. Health Begins. March 24, 2022. Available at: https://healthbegins.org/cone-health-greensboro-housing. Accessed August 29, 2022.
4. Philanthropic Initiative for Racial Equity. Grantmaking with a racial justice lens. Available at: https://racialequity.org/grantmaking-with-a-racial-justice-lens. Accessed August 29, 2022.

2

Collaborating for Success: The Symbiotic Relationship Between Communities and Institutions

James Bell III, DSW, and Jodi Cunningham, PhD

Regardless of where we sit, most of us want the same things from our communities—to work well, to be safe from violence and illness, and to thrive. As public health service providers and decision makers, we ensure that these goals are embedded in the culture of our organizations and programs and want them to serve as a critical bridge that connects our organizations and programs to communities. The reality is that we cannot foster the communities we aspire to have if we are working in silos. Collaborative partnerships serve as a powerful way to improve community conditions by working together to solve problems that are bigger than any one of us. We do this by engaging our communities.

As aspirational as our vision for communities is and the corresponding partnerships necessary to bring them to life are, community engagement as a conduit for change does not always allow for full participation of the community from start to finish. Organizations may seek to engage the community, but red tape, organizational policies, and the inability to "meet people where they are" often prevent full participation and ownership from those with the highest stakes.

One example is an inequitable infrastructure that exists in organizations and their relationships with vendors. Oftentimes, even though an organization's mission may align with supporting smaller and minority-owned businesses for partnerships and contracts, policies may prevent this work because those smaller organizations may not meet certain insurance requirements that larger organizations are able to meet, thereby creating more risk. When this occurs, it is often the result of endeavors that were more transactional in nature or that typically benefit only one party (most often our institutions). To achieve deeper, more meaningful, and sustainable community engagement, communities and institutions must work together every step of the way to reimagine what is possible. Authentic and intentional relationships between the two must be built on trust and can

> Community engagement increases visibility and understanding of issues while empowering communities to have more influence over the decisions that affect their daily lives.

When working with a community, we must be flexible, using values and principles to guide the work as opposed to a checklist of things that should be done. Our organizations are typically guided by rules and regulations that don't translate well to community work. Therefore, it is imperative we focus on relationships as a vehicle for meeting our mutually established goals.

offer a strategic platform for collaboration. These components are essential to advancing health equity, transforming the way we provide services, and shifting the way individuals experience their communities and our institutions.

Such collaboration requires the involvement of multiple partners, each with its own complex histories that can make engagement work particularly challenging. If the goal is to truly work *with* communities and not to work *on behalf* of communities, we find ourselves in a position to build capacity by supporting community-led solutions. In particular, instances of exploitation and manipulation are barriers to advancing the work and must be resolved early in the process of collaboration. This could entail allocating resources so that members can be active participants and identifying community interests and goals.

Lessons Learned

Here we highlight a few of the lessons learned when it comes to collaboration to support community engagement from Avondale Children Thrive (ACT), a cross-sector collaboration designed to improve maternal and child health, as an avenue to decrease infant mortality among families in the Avondale neighborhood, located in Cincinnati, Ohio (for more on Avondale Children Thrive, see: https://buildhealthchallenge.org/communities/2-avondale-children-thrive). As members of a cross-sector collaboration between housing, health care, and public health partners, all ACT collaborators colead with neighborhood Health Champions, which is a hired housing-based team of resident leaders. Health Champions are well-liked, caring, and trusting neighbors who are invested in the growth and success of their community. Every community has these natural leaders, yet communities lack the social infrastructure to support their leadership. In Avondale, ACT changed that by bringing structure, supports, training, and continued technical assistance to ensure that these leaders will have the power and community stand they need to create community change.

Unlike other community health initiatives, ACT began in the middle of a $29.5 million neighborhood transformation in 2012, thanks to a Choice Neighborhoods Implementation (CNI) grant from the Department of Housing and Urban Development to The Community Builders, a nonprofit affordable housing organization. The CNI grant

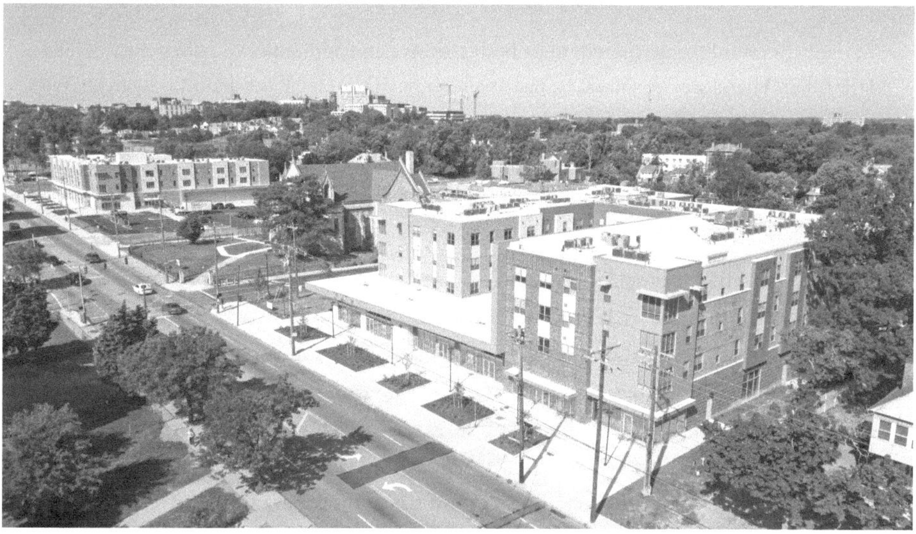

Source: Reprinted with permission from The Community Builders.

Figure 2-1. Avondale Town Center

allowed for the renovation and new construction of affordable housing (319 total units) while also redeveloping the business center hub, bringing much needed and community-informed amenities, including a laundromat, a Federally Qualified Health Center, a daycare, a social justice center, and a grocery store—the first in the neighborhood after over a decade (see Figure 2-1, Avondale Town Center). A key pillar of the CNI grant was to support residents to maintain housing stability and receive wraparound social services and connections to resources as part of the transformation. In 2018, The Community Builders together with Cincinnati Children's Hospital and Cincinnati Health Department leveraged the resource allocations and transformation happening in the community to seek funding from The BUILD Health Challenge (BUILD) to support and mobilize residents and community partners to create a healthy Avondale for families to thrive by combining one-on-one peer support with more systemic change.

Lesson 1: Bring Your Most Authentic Self and Lay the Groundwork for Authentic Partners.

As collaborators, how we show up for our communities will set the tone for how communities will work together with us moving forward. It is commonplace to want to drive decision-making—leading every step of the way—but this can further marginalize groups and limit their opportunity to participate equitably. Being intentional suggests we develop relationships with communities and their members to develop a mutual

> We want community engagement to be both effective and authentic, knowing one can lead to the other. Therefore, we should be just as authentic as we expect the community to be. We must move from merely informing the community about decisions we've made to creating partnerships.

purpose and benefit for engagement. All our decisions and actions should be part of an effort to foster more trust with community members. The only way to do this is to take the time needed to understand differences and find commonalities. To this end, we practice active listening to uncover key concerns and rarely heard voices. Much of the level-setting is to recognize the different kinds of groups we are working with and to create the foundation for collaboration.

Creating this kind of shift then allows community members to be active participants in creating the healthy residences they want while fostering more trust with our institutions as the backbone. This work requires accepting the uncertainty, risk, and openness to divergent ideas that can challenge us and make us uncomfortable. When it comes to resident engagement, even the most well-meaning institution can be hesitant to lean into discomfort. For those engaged in true systems change initiatives, there must be space for explicit discussions of race and equity, as well as how our institutionalized structures frequently support inequity.

In building relationships with the community, we must treat community members as authentic partners. We at ACT found success in hiring community members to serve on the team, providing space and time for residents to be at every table consistently and compensating members for their time and expertise. We also found that not all money is good money. In hiring residents who live in subsidized housing or are on fixed incomes, we learned to carefully consider the amount of the stipend given for the community members' work, so as to not inflict the "cliff effect." The cliff effect occurs when an increase of income contributes to a loss of public benefits and yet is not enough of an increase to positively change someone's economic status so they no longer need such benefits. With ACT, we set monthly volunteer stipends at $200, as anything above that amount fully counts as income and could increase a volunteer's rent, threatening that individual's economic security.

In pursuing authenticity, we also learned to tailor our interventions. Leading with community meant supporting individuals with their needs, and not implementing one-size-fits-all initiatives. Some of the Health Champion leaders had additional employment or were working toward full-time employment; thus, they already had income to report to the property manager, and the additional volunteer stipend funding would not negatively change their economic situation. In this case, some team members were willing to work a few more hours a month to gain increased stipends.

> If you are not a member of the community you seek to serve, your understanding of that community is limited.

Thankfully, the ACT leadership team was able to effectively create an environment where the health team was able to discuss wages in an open format, providing critique of structures and offering solutions. Although this is a critical piece of balancing power, the most important part is what that leadership then chooses to do with the information. These types of conversations are where trust is either built or crumbles.

Lesson 2: Power Can Make or Break the Relationship.

As practitioners, within organizations, with access to broader collaboratives and capital, we hold significant power. To achieve the goals shared by our organizations and communities, we must rethink what it means to redistribute that power. And this can be uncomfortable if the partners have not discussed shared decision-making according to power differentials.

All community engagement initiatives must begin by acknowledging and confronting the unavoidable power dynamics at play. Power relationships between institutions and community members are constantly being negotiated both formally and informally. In our various spaces, even something as commonly overlooked as jargon can drive gaps in accessibility for community members. Terms like "concentrated areas of poverty" or "low-opportunity areas" create a deficit-oriented frame and can make it difficult to fully engage. Gleaning from the work of the Health Champions in Avondale, we found that hiring and equipping neighborhood leaders with important health information and providing access to health partners was a shining success in community engagement, in particular embodying "meeting people where they are" (see Figure 2-2, The Poinciana). In some ways, the fact that this initiative involved housing created an environment for the acceleration of progress and trust building. Relationships between Health Champions and residents seemed to be stronger than they would have been had we hired team members from outside the neighborhood. There was, for instance,

> When we encounter situations that challenge our comfort levels or the status quo within our organizations and partnerships, we must pause to ask ourselves a few questions: Who seems most powerful in this context, and why? What type of power are we and others bringing to this partnership? What are the influences that could change the power structure in our partnership? All involved in the partnership must identify opportunities for transparent discussions of power.

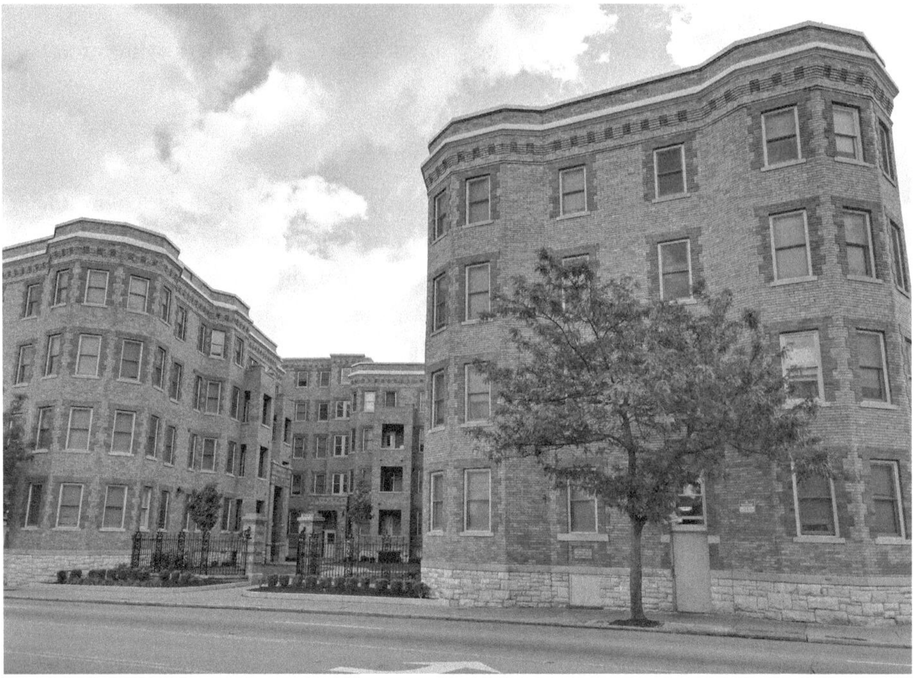

Source: Reprinted with permission from The Community Builders.

Figure 2-2. The Poinciana

a genuine understanding between women when discussing the challenges and trauma of neighborhood violence. Yet in other ways, Health Champions being immersed in housing served to deter some residents from engaging with us. Some residents felt that the Health Champions were "too close to home," since in their aim to support healthy and stable housing for all residents they coordinated and worked so closely with The Community Builders property management team. There was fear, alongside a historical context that for some residents screamed "do not trust." We fully realized that Avondale was not a monolith and that prioritizing the individual needs and concerns of mothers was the only way forward.

After acknowledging such power dynamics, we must be equipped to share and, in some cases, relinquish that power. Loosening the grip of control suggests we consider the benefits of shared decision-making and identify mutual goals. We must ask ourselves, for example, Who makes decisions about sustainability and future grant writing to sustain nonprofit work? Does the community have a say in which type of funding awards to try to secure? In the nonprofit world, we oftentimes operate in a rushed and underresourced fashion, especially within the current landscape of philanthropy and vying for dollars for needed community programs. This can create situations wherein leaders make decisions about the direction of a community initiative without ever consulting the community in question or considering the correct weight of community feelings. Making decisions about funding and sustainability at the leadership level is a quick-fix approach, but it ignores community input. Although the systems may not support the expediency needed to develop competitive proposals, finding ways to engage members of the community and bring them into the sustainability and funding process is important. We have historically used top-down decision-making only to inform residents, resulting in further distance between communities and institutions. Resisting the urge to use a quick-fix top-down approach demonstrates our willingness to be collaborative partners and instills trust in community members.

Lesson 3: Be Accountable and Transparent.

Authentic community engagement is the foundation for deeper, stronger, and more trusting relationships between our institutions and communities. We are called to be clear and open about all our processes, including the range of views and ideas expressed. Residents who are shut out of strategic and decision-making processes often end up feeling disempowered and unmotivated. Although it can feel like another meeting on the calendar, we should have regular check-ins to gauge progress, seek feedback on our process, and generate new ideas grounded on community concerns. These informal moments can yield opportunities that reveal root causes to the problems we are looking to address or connections we want to make for sustainability.

To be accountable means we must be proactive. When information is being made available or a decision must be made, we must be equipped to share. Community members may not know what information is necessary or relevant, given the issue, and we should not expect them to seek out the details. Even in moments of crisis when all the facts are not yet available, we can share what we do know and follow up with additional information as soon as it is available. This approach includes open access to essential information such as how our institutions operate and perform—and when we fail to perform as we should. It is our responsibility to ensure the community has access to information and understands the implications for said information. We cannot suppress details that would make us look bad. We should establish clear transparency guidelines in collaboration with our partners, even if there are consequences to the way we as an institution are perceived.

> Community engagement and its decision-making cannot be considered transparent if important voices—that is, voices from the community—are overlooked, disregarded, or dismissed. Engagement efforts must therefore be an honest and complete accounting of facts and context essential to ensuring informed and equitable participation and decision-making.

Lesson 4: Seek Out the Strengths.

Every resident, young or old, has unique individual talents, experiences, beliefs, and values. While we know there is value in each person's contributions, we must also recognize, appreciate, and leverage their strengths. In return, participants will know that you and your organization understand and see the many ways in which their participation is helpful and important. Our initiatives absolutely must build on the assets and power already found in the community such as historical knowledge of the community, which is information that only those deeply immersed in neighborhood relationships would know, and individual skills, comprising expertise and approaches to solving complex community issues, which are most often found by those most affected. Although the ACT resident champion position was created as a one-on-one coaching role, the leadership team found that some Health Champions had strengths in other areas, such as advocacy and policy engagement, so they revised the job description to reflect the Health Champions' strengths.

The strengths perspective leverages aspirations rather than focuses on problems and deficits. After expanding the Health Champions' roles, we saw team members working together, fully rooted in their passions. Our coaching Health Champions worked to discuss the benefits of breastfeeding with mothers, for example. However, in discussion the team revealed that the neighborhood community was not supportive of women breastfeeding in public, which also contributed to the narrative that mothers weren't breastfeeding at all. Because of the cross-sector collaboration and unique funding award for the Health Champion initiative, the Health Champion team was able to work together with the Cincinnati Health Department to draft, advocate for, and successfully pass a breastfeeding-friendly policy in 23 City of Cincinnati recreation centers. By working together and leveraging one another's strengths, we were able to increase trust between organizational and community partners while also maintaining the community and institution relationship. When everyone plays their part, while keeping the community at center, we are able to achieve these neighborhood-level changes on a larger, more replicable scale.

> Every community and those working in it are going to face problems or unmet needs, and when faced with such a challenge it is important to respond by building on what is already working.

What the Future Holds

By engaging communities, institutions can advance sustainable programs that place the focus on people and opportunities that make it possible for them to thrive. Our efforts

> The underlying belief behind community engagement initiatives is that people affected by a problem have the best solutions. They bring lived experience to our systems and processes that cannot be learned elsewhere and when combined with organizational knowledge and resources create partnerships that are more innovative and likely to lead to desired outcomes.

should aspire to create a sense of ownership within the community, a key factor for future change initiatives. When discussing the renovations and opening of the community town center, the late Dr. Anita Brentley, a key public health champion of the Avondale community, shared that "Avondale residents just wanted to put a brick in the wall." She further explained that they wanted to be a part of the transformation. They wanted co-ownership by way of giving their opinions and ideas and then seeing them reflected in the development happening around them. The Community Builders is committed to recognizing and honoring Dr. Brentley's vision of integrating resident voices and ownership as a key pillar of neighborhood transformation.

Strong partnerships with communities should result in mutual investment—whether financial or social—and should create a sense of buy-in and shared ownership that extends beyond a grant period. Institutions, individual residents, businesses, and even policymakers cannot act alone to create and sustain healthy communities. Many leaders recognize the need to collaborate across sectors and with communities in our engagement processes and already do so. With ACT, we have found that engaging communities in a variety of ways has had numerous positive results, not only at the individual level but at neighborhood levels too. It has increased the community's understanding and appreciation of public health, helped us to build trust and credibility between our partners and our residents, and facilitated genuine involvement that has traditionally been absent from the decision-making process. We are excited to continue testing, refining, and sharing our work and power with communities as we tackle future disparities.

As communities catalyze new networks of relationships and find new problem-solving methods and new inclusive decision-making spaces, our institutions have the opportunity to serve as the backbone for a more equitable future. And that is not without its share of challenges. Experience tells us that trust is not easily built and that mistrust is not easily reversed. The process of collaboration, in particular for institutions and communities, is an ongoing one that is constantly evolving as the actors evolve. Navigating these relationships requires our commitment to horizontal power structures and prioritizing collaboration. Ultimately, the end goals aren't just the outcomes of the initiative itself but the connections that emerge—and endure—between partners.

3

Centering Community Engagement

Jessica Mulcahy, MA, and Emily Yu, MBA

When fully realized, community engagement becomes a powerful North Star for an organization or a team, informing their strategies and guiding their practices. In previous chapters, key terms, definitions, and stories have laid the groundwork for a fundamental understanding of what community engagement is and its importance to public health efforts. This level-setting provides some of the core concepts and tools related to how public health practitioners can more effectively engage with community members as well as establishes the importance of recognizing the inherent power and expertise community members already hold.

And while this context is critically important in our efforts to drive sustainable improvements in community health and health equity, the reality is that no one framework, case study, or toolkit will ever be able to offer us a step-by-step solution to addressing a community's health disparities and ensuring that all its residents have the opportunity to thrive.

Public health practitioners know better than most that there is an urgent need to facilitate and amplify community-centered efforts—not only to remove economic and social obstacles to health but also to dismantle barriers to equity and build up new pathways that offer redress for historical inequities. This multipronged approach, nested within a community-centered effort, is the necessary on-ramp to change if we want communities to have the opportunity to truly thrive.

It is in this spirit that we invite readers to explore community-centered approaches that advance health equity as an opportunity for dynamic change, ultimately transforming the internal working culture of their team or organization as well as potentially influencing and informing the approaches of their partners. To gain clarity on these fundamental issues, we challenge you to consider the following:

- Your current perspectives on the why, the who, and the how of community engagement.
- The need to reimagine the ways in which you want, and perhaps need, to evolve your approaches.
- What it means to center community voice as a public health practitioner within an organization.
- What possibilities might exist if "centering community" is adopted as a core value within your organization.

> The real opportunity for public health practitioners is in the act of centering community, in bringing forth a mindset shift among those involved that prioritizes community, and in changing policies and practices that will ultimately help build power among community members.

To help you and other public health practitioners navigate this process, this chapter provides readers with the opportunity to think through what community engagement means to them, to center their core values of engagement and equity, and to explore using those essential building blocks to center community voice within an organization (see Box 3-1).

Box 3-1. Key Frameworks for Engagement

There is a key distinction between understanding community engagement and operationalizing it in one's efforts to improve population health. While there is no one-size-fits-all solution when it comes to the practice of community engagement, these frameworks, and others like them, provide a generalized map to guide engagement work and provide the overarching wise practices gleaned from others who have gone down this path before you. These have been curated to highlight two concepts that can help you better center community engagement in your own efforts and that of your organization: understanding power dynamics and key considerations for early engagement work.

1. Thinking through power dynamics: A variety of frameworks for engagement offer ways of understanding the relationship between the organization and the community in terms of how they interact. Commonly used frameworks include the following:

    - International Association for Public Participation (IAP2) Spectrum of Participation (see Figure 3-1): https://www.iap2.org.
    - Davidson's Wheel of Empowerment: https://www.researchgate.net/figure/The-wheel-of-participation-Source-adapted-from-Davidson-41_fig2_51834104.
    - Arnstein's Ladder of Citizen Participation: https://www.citizenshandbook.org/arnsteinsladder.html.

2. Key considerations for engagement efforts: Checklists and worksheets are tools that are useful for carrying out early engagement work and for helping others understand what is involved. Examples of these include:

    - King County's Community Engagement Worksheet: https://kingcounty.gov/elected/executive/equity-social-justice/tools-resources.aspx.
    - PolicyLink's Community Engagement Checklist: https://www.policylink.org/sites/default/files/COMMUNITY%20ENGAGEMENT%20CHECKLIST.pdf.
    - Centers for Disease Control and Prevention's Meaningful Community Engagement for Health and Equity Guide: https://www.cdc.gov/nccdphp/dnpao/health-equity/health-equity-guide/pdf/health-equity-guide/Health-Equity-Guide-sect-1-2.pdf.

Naming and framing the operational and historical aspects of community engagement and detangling some of the core power dynamics inherent in a relationship in which community is involved are critical first steps. Frameworks and guides, such as the ones we have referenced, represent just a handful of what is available to you and serve as useful safety nets in conceptualizing what is in essence a dynamic and ever-changing process. The next important step occurs when these tools are tailored for a specific purpose and context. The best way to do that effectively is in partnership with the community.

INCREASING IMPACT ON THE DECISION →

	INFORM	CONSULT	INVOLVE	COLLABORATE	EMPOWER
PUBLIC PARTICIPATION GOAL	To provide the public with balanced and objective information to assist them in understanding the problem, alternatives, opportunities and/or solutions.	To obtain public feedback on analysis, alternatives and/or decisions.	To work directly with the public throughout the process to ensure that public concerns and aspirations are consistently understood and considered.	To partner with the public in each aspect of the decision including the development of alternatives and the identification of the preferred solution.	To place final decision making in the hands of the public.
PROMISE TO THE PUBLIC	We will keep you informed.	We will keep you informed, listen to and acknowledge concerns and aspirations, and provide feedback on how public input influenced the decision.	We will work with you to ensure that your concerns and aspirations are directly reflected in the alternatives developed and provide feedback on how public input influenced the decision.	We will look to you for advice and innovation in formulating solutions and incorporate your advice and recommendations into the decisions to the maximum extent possible.	We will implement what you decide.

Source: Reprinted with permission of IAP2 ©International Association for Public Participation www.iap2.org.[1]
Note: IAP2's Spectrum of Public Participation was designed to assist with the selection of the level of participation that defines the public's role in any public participation process. The Spectrum is used internationally, and it is found in public participation plans around the world.

Figure 3-1. International Association for Public Participation (IAP2) Spectrum of Public Participation

REIMAGINING YOUR WHY

Do you have clarity of purpose when it comes to engaging with community? Do you understand what you intend to do and what you have the power to do? In other words, when it comes to community engagement, the intent (why), the people (who), and the process (how) of engagement are all equally as important as the outcome (what). While both concepts—community engagement and community-centered approaches—rely on people in communities and, in most cases, people with lived experience in the issues or conditions at the center of the effort, the approaches are fundamentally different.* Being clear on which type of strategy an organization wants to follow and understanding why it is important not only for effectively communicating with community members but also for building a culture of transparency and trust among partners are critical considerations.

- Organization-centered community engagement: Even when used in the context of a long-term strategy, this approach is often applied in more tactical ways and is used for the benefit of moving an organization's agenda forward, sometimes with guidance or

* "People with lived experience" is defined here as those who have direct experience with the key issues being addressed.

direction from the community. For example, one might carry out a community engagement strategy to build relationships with a group of residents for input or decision-making related to a project or program.

- Community-centered processes: These processes draw on residents' power and decision-making rather than necessarily improving an organization's efforts. It is held as a value that is actively practiced, informing how the organization works, the focus of its efforts, and the ongoing role that community members play in determining the focus and direction of the effort.

An organization must decide up front which approach it is taking. Once the stance of the organization is clear, it is possible to understand what is in your power to do and move things forward accordingly. A single staff member cannot take on a community-centered approach if the organization is generally focused on an organization-centered engagement strategy. Such a change requires an examination of power dynamics, organizational readiness, and identification of organizational stakeholders and decision makers. In addition, such a shift would require an understanding of what the organization's commitment to a community-centered approach might be and how that would shift the focus of the organization's work.

To help ground you in evaluating your why when it comes to engagement and centering community, consider the following question: *How can lived experience help frame solutions and disrupt systems that have caused racial inequities?* This prompt by stakeholders of The BUILD Health Challenge (BUILD), a national awards program supporting community-driven, cross-sector partnerships advancing health equity, was posed during a recent listening tour that included practitioners from public health departments, community-based organizations (CBOs), hospitals, and resident groups. BUILD used this prompt and ensuing conversations to shift power in the development and facilitation of the listening tour from funders and the organizing body to community awardees. The listening tour was designed to bring community voice into the design of a new funding round of BUILD and to authentically center it on racial equity.

Three key observations surfaced during the listening tour that help articulate why community engagement and centering community are fundamental to one's health efforts.[2]

1. Institutional power can be given or shared, but communities already have power: There are two fundamental paths for considering power. The first is framed as institutions and other decision-making bodies having power, and that part of the work is about taking that power for a community to wield in favor of community-driven priorities. The other is that communities already have power and it must only be realized and focused, rather than ceded by an institution, to achieve change. The BUILD experience provided an opportunity for CBOs, with their resident-led approaches and connections, to recognize that they held real power and did not

need it to be "given" to them by their hospital, health plan, or public health department partners.

2. Centering community is an ongoing commitment to keep community voice at the foundation of the work: To center community, and to do so meaningfully, often requires both internal and external changes to occur that speak to the mission of an organization, the goals of a project, and the values of a community. Changes that go beyond the literal interpretation, where community members are "present," must instead involve community participation from the beginning on prioritization, design, implementation, and learning. Depending on the organization, this approach may require changes to organizational policies and practices, an ability to name and shift power dynamics, and changes to organizational values.
3. Centering racial equity is an effective catalyst for change: Placing racial equity at the core of the work enables the group to identify and tackle root causes of an issue and to create an intentional space for understanding the context and history of the community as a necessary part of the work. This results in a deeper understanding of what the priorities of the effort should be and helps to identify what systems, processes, and norms need to be put in place to address the historical inequities perpetuated by existing structures. It is very difficult, if not impossible, to get to the who or the how without acknowledging that this is a core component of the work and centering community.

The process, which began as a basic listening tour, grew into a pathway for a much more robust and dynamic form of engagement. The learnings, including these three insights, when acted on, helped BUILD stakeholders codesign a roadmap to reimagine this health equity funding program's focus, criteria, and implementation structure by considering what was possible, not just what could be different. Also important is to consider what remains unspoken or unaccounted for in this engagement (see Box 3-2).

Box 3-2. Reflection Question: What Remains Unspoken or Unaccounted for in Your Conversations About Community Engagement?

Discussions involving community engagement and the centering of community are often challenging because they require acknowledgment of power imbalances and historical and/or ongoing discrimination, as well as social and racial injustices that have contributed to the need for greater engagement. Yet at the same time, such conversations, fueled by an authentic willingness to collaborate in support of a better and healthier community, can be effective vehicles for change. Public health leaders in particular may want to consider putting their team and organizational support behind local efforts that intentionally focus on building relationships as the necessary first step for challenging conversations and innovative solutions related to identified community issues. Starting with trust in the form of proven partnerships can ultimately help shed light on the "unspoken" challenges the community faces, strengthen and improve collaborative programmatic efforts over time, and highlight new ways of thinking about addressing challenges traditional partners had not considered.

REIMAGINING YOUR WHO

How are you sharing power and considering identity when it comes to identifying your team, your partners, and others who are part of your efforts to engage with community? Attempting to identify who represents a community is a critical, yet often challenging component of any community-centered collaboration effort. For some, the answer may mean working with a local CBO, with individuals experiencing homelessness, or with the volunteers at the local farmers market. Or it may mean forging a new relationship with a group you do not know. Rarely does it mean involving every single community member or relying on just one to two residents to represent an entire community. Ultimately, what matters is prioritizing those in the community who are or who have been most affected by the issue(s) being addressed.

Community engagement starts by recognizing the inherent power, knowledge, and aspirations that exist within communities and also their ability to drive sustainable improvements across sectors and issues. For those who traditionally hold power and resources, such as public health departments, private sector entities, and funders, this understanding also recognizes that they alone cannot solve these systemic challenges without community (as we have defined it). For example, communities participating in BUILD are required to have a CBO leading each community collaboration. The intent is to help shift the balance of power in favor of the community while also aligning with those entities that may have significant resources or may benefit from existing power structures—such as the local public health department, hospital, or health plan—each of which is required by BUILD to be a partner in a collaborative.

By working together with the CBO as the lead partner and recipient of the BUILD award, each collaborative is encouraged to cultivate a cross-sector and community-centered partnership. Participants noted that this arrangement was successful in paving the way for changes in authority, decision-making, and leadership among the partners.[1] And whereas a rebalancing of power did occur in many cases, participants reflected that the inclusion of a CBO as an intermediary and facilitator for the community could not substitute for or replace the sharing of power, the centering of racial justice, or the process of cocreation within the program.[2] Such systemic changes ultimately required the shifting of power, both explicit and implicit, with the express goal of building community power. Those who achieved such shifts did so by building and reinforcing trust among the partners through transparency, feedback loops, and consistency that manifests only in groups that have worked together and built trust with one another over time.

As public health department leaders serving in the community, you play an important role not only in supporting *community representation* but also in laying the groundwork for this shift in power to drive authentic *community engagement*. It is important to question how lived experience in the context of our programs, organizations,

Box 3-3. Reflection Question: Who Is Missing?

A fundamental concept throughout this chapter is the idea that no one individual, organization, or team can create the type of transformative change we seek in health. Use this opportunity to review the team and partners with which you are working. What is each person's role? Now think with that group about the change you are collectively trying to make and what it will take to be realized. Are any individuals or organizational stakeholders missing from your team?

- If yes, ask yourself why. What obstacles or past relationship history might need to be addressed in order to change this? What might need to change about the way your engagement strategy is currently constructed to center community voices in the effort?
- If no, and you already have the stakeholders you need working with you, confirm that team members each understand their role as well as the power dynamics between one another. Do others on the team share the same understanding?

and partnerships is being lifted up and used to frame solutions.* How is centering community strategically and intentionally disrupting the systems that have caused and sustain racial inequities? And who may be missing from your team (see Box 3-3)?

REIMAGINING YOUR HOW: THE PRACTICE OF ENGAGING COMMUNITY AND COMMUNITY-CENTERED APPROACHES

When considering community engagement and centering it in one's organizational values, strategies, and approaches, it is important to understand not only the why and the who but also the how—namely, how you and your team will honor and also operationalize that commitment. When you are designing, implementing, or making sense of outcomes from a programmatic effort or strategy, be mindful that centering community programmatically, particularly paying heed to the voices of people with lived experience, can help ensure that the effort is perceived as a prioritized need within the community and that it is designed in ways that make sense in the context of that community.

At the beginning, taking a learning approach in understanding what community means is key. This includes giving yourself and others the time to understand the context of the community, to listen to a variety of voices and perspectives, and to create a transparent environment for engagement. In order to carry out these initial steps, it is often helpful to engage additional facilitation support, reach out to existing

*In naming and placing value on one's experiences in relation to an issue, we must also remember that the term "lived experience" is being used as a classification and descriptor, not as a monolith. This idea captures the varied and diverse representation of a community's members and their personal experiences. It is in this diversity of person and place that we can begin to understand the concept of one's lived experience and its relation to the identity of the community.

resident leadership networks such as community health workers or *promotoras**, and spend time in various parts of the community to get to know people and begin to build relationships.

Centering community voice authentically can, over time, help build a relationship based on trust between formal organizations and community members. Authentic relationships are ones built on transparency, following the values espoused, and honoring the intent of the work. Trust between partners is the foundation for most open conversation about who needs to be at the table, whether that includes additional formal organizations and institutions or new groups of community residents representing subcommunities.

You should also recognize community members who are closest to the issues you are trying to address as the context experts that they are, given their lived experience. Doing so may mean acknowledging the value of their experiences, providing compensation commensurate with their efforts, and/or sharing power in understanding and making decisions related to the issue at hand. Most important is to create relationships with community members and other local partners on the basis of a shared commitment to the community or a shared value, not a specific project. This framework will help you create more effective opportunities and sustainable strategies in support of your shared goals.

By centering community from the beginning, you can ensure that your work can be truly beneficial to people with lived experience and those who are most affected by the issues you are confronting. Doing this also ensures greater potential for this effort to be sustained over the long term. And because ongoing listening and refinement by community residents is at the center, the effort will be better able to evolve as shifts in who lives in a community and other changes occur in the long term.

Taking time to develop this understanding of the community and one's organization requires patience. These practices lay the foundation for understanding how to approach community engagement and determining whether a community-centered approach is feasible for your organization. This process will also help you identify any existing networks of people ready to engage, bring to light existing engagement efforts by other entities, and help you and your team better understand what types of engagement will best position residents to use their inherent power collectively.

Although the temptation might be strong to get to work implementing changes, do not fall into the trap of jumping right into program planning without first acknowledging what it will take to address existing power imbalances and how the group participants can work together to build power within the community. Taking the time and allocating the resources for this step will ultimately help strengthen and ground the team with a

---

*Promotoras, or Promotores de Salud, is the Spanish term for "Community Health Workers." For more information on Promotores de Salud, visit: https://www.cdc.gov/minorityhealth/promotores/index.html.

The wide variety of ways to engage is both exciting and daunting at the same time when we recognize that there is no one "right" path to take. Rather, it is the journey we take together as partners with a shared goal that ultimately builds power, deepens trust, and lays the foundation for transformative change to happen within a community.

unifying perspective that can help participants overcome the twists and turns inherent in such efforts.

Finally, let's discuss how centering community in health equity efforts enables community partners to better identify pathways for doing so and consider key questions that need to be addressed along the way. Throughout the listening tour, participants shared that they were in various places along the community engagement journey (even partners working within the same collaborative, within a given community, were in different places), but all recognized that there was a trajectory toward equity and community voice-centered efforts. Participants in BUILD's listening tour articulated that power sharing is essential, and it goes well beyond traditional community engagement tactics. A diverse set of people with lived experiences must become equal decision-making partners, and institutions must yield their power. Figuring out how to set conditions for power sharing, however, can be elusive.

In addition to this external work, a prerequisite of authentic engagement is understanding and being transparent about the intentions, motivations, and time commitment of the organization one is affiliated with. Having a clear picture of these factors and knowing how to navigate internally in your organization are essential for building strong relationships with community members. Also important is to understand your own power and position within an organization so that you are able at the outset to articulate what you have the power to do within and on behalf of your organization. In other words, when it comes to community engagement, the intent (why), the people (who), and the process (how) of engagement are all equally as important as the outcome (what). Consider also the long-term implications of your work (see Box 3-4).

Box 3-4. Reflection Question: What Are the Long-Term Implications of Your Efforts?

Starting with your shared strategy and the approach you are taking for the work being done, ask yourself if this foundation was created in collaboration with those in the community most greatly affected by the issue at hand. In what way(s) is this approach being defined and put into practice so that it supports the building of resident capacity, in the process fostering learning and establishing trust and accountability? How will this effort not only support the shifting of power to the community but also better enable the community to hold power and use it most effectively as a long-term proposition?

A JOURNEY, NOT A DESTINATION

The study of community engagement is one that is well documented and well worn by practitioners across sectors. Despite the numerous frameworks, case studies, and examples referenced in this chapter, the reality is that it's still not enough when it comes to engagement that advances better health for all. It's not enough to rightsize the power imbalances that keep decision-making out of the hands of residents. It's not enough to dismantle the systems that perpetuate and disenfranchise those who may be most impacted by an issue. And it's not enough to change prevailing narratives that control one's story and decide how it is told.

It is incumbent on each and every one of us to stop to consider the intersectionality of community engagement and the centering of community. Let's reimagine how these two concepts show up and manifest in our work, and let's envision the impact on communities as a result. We must question the why, the who, and the how so that we do not simply engage community but rather center community and, in so doing, foster the mindset shift needed to advance health equity.

As stewards of change, we must accept that our understanding of community engagement and practice of centering community will always be a work in progress—and that's a good thing. For just as our communities are dynamic and ever-evolving entities, so too are the challenges and opportunities we face within them. There is no ready-made template when it comes to community engagement, no proverbial finish line to cross, and no checklist to complete where once done we can claim our work is complete. It is up to us to help communities write the next chapter of our shared story.

Meaningful community engagement takes time, patience, and consistency. With a laser focus on deepening community engagement, demonstrated over time, you and your partners can strengthen your relationship with one another and foster trust with members of the broader community. That is reimagining the "what" of this work and the objective we all must strive for. Just as with equity, it is the individual moments of progress on engagement that become interdependent over time, eventually weaving together the change to create the groundwork for a new norm. Much like the push and pull of gravity, we can never capture it per se, but we can learn to lean into and work with its powerful force.

> To achieve such a transformative change in community health requires us as public health champions to also change our own policies, practices, and funding streams and how we collectively think about community.

REFERENCES

1. International Association for Public Participation. IAP2 spectrum of public participation. Available at: https://cdn.ymaws.com/www.iap2.org/resource/resmgr/pillars/Spectrum_8.5x11_Print.pdf. Accessed October 4, 2022.
2. The BUILD Health Challenge. Listening, learning, and leading together: insights from The BUILD Health Challenge's 2021 listening tour. November 2021. Available at: https://buildhealthchallenge.org/resources/builds-2021-listening-tour-report. Accessed September 9, 2022.

4

What Does Good Community Engagement Design Look, Sound, and Feel Like?

Evette De Luca

Those who are closest to the issues are closest to the solutions.

–Community Wealth Partners[1]

We live in an era of competing, complex discomforts—today's social complexities, including those involving public health, call for the cocreation of power and health strategies to transform communities. Those who are closest to the social issues we seek to combat must play critical leadership roles to ensure authentic engagement and to sustain collective attention. In addition, public health departments and public health leaders have unprecedented opportunities not only to enact change but also to adopt, invest in, and fund an often overlooked component of this transformation work: effective storytelling that creates the narrative for the change. By doing so, we can engage communities, lift the veil of invisibility that may shroud vulnerable people, tap into upstream solutions, fuel positive systems change, and learn even as we fail forward together (see Figure 4-1).

In many ways, it has never been easier to engage communities and create storytelling platforms in the hyperconnected social world we inhabit. TikTok, Instagram, Facebook, YouTube, WhatsApp: through these five major streaming services, we are subject to a multitude of exponentially unfolding stories, a constant search, creation, and control of "truth." Modern media-driven communication, with social media at the helm, amplifies ideas, generates meaning, and drives conflict. When it comes to authoring and controlling narratives, communities often lose. Our content-obsessed culture has changed the battlefield from that of a war over "hearts and minds" to that of "minds and eyeballs." Traditional power holders, like large brands and marketing firms (think PepsiCo),

> As champions of community health, we must ask ourselves, What does it look like to put important public health ideas into effective crowdsourcing action through community voices? And, How can we most effectively cut through the competing noise generated through social media so that effective public health storytelling can permeate our sector's atmosphere or specific community atmospheres in effective ways?

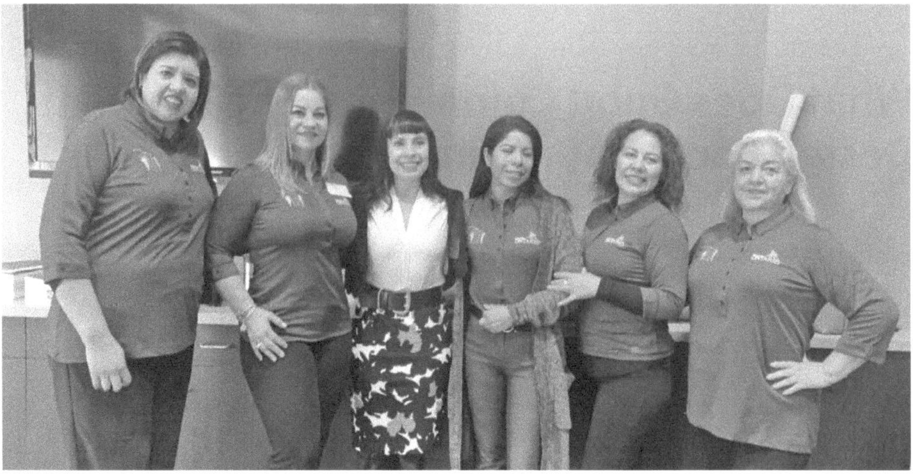

Source: Reprinted with permission of Social Impact Artists.

Figure 4-1. Social Impact Artists and Healthy Ontario Resident Leaders

ply the internet with memes and messaging. How can communities, especially vulnerable communities, compete to lead their own narratives?

These social media mechanisms stoke and feed an appetite for populist, viral storytelling, creating unparalleled channels of engagement. They have also resulted in a bombardment of stories about danger, disillusionment, and disenfranchisement, by those who benefit from the continuation of such narratives—and which ultimately make public health leadership more complex. These dynamics played out during the greatest public health crisis of modern times and show no sign of disappearing. The answer begins with community members using their own media channels to provide their truth, to become the "influencers," and in so doing helping to dismantle the "media halo" that controls public health narratives.[2]

Public Health's Role in Shaping the Story of Community Health

Storytelling has become an increasingly valuable tool for public health practitioners to use when communicating complex or critical health information to the public because of its ability to punch with emotion, create connection, and enhance comprehension—it is a skill and tool that are no longer optional. And far from being "empty vessels" needing to be filled with information, community members can be strong allies in engagement and storytelling strategies. Consider the pain, burnout, bewilderment, and numbness we have experienced during the COVID-19 pandemic and what we will continue to experience in its wake. More effective public health storytelling may shift the culture of fear, misinformation, disinformation, and panic

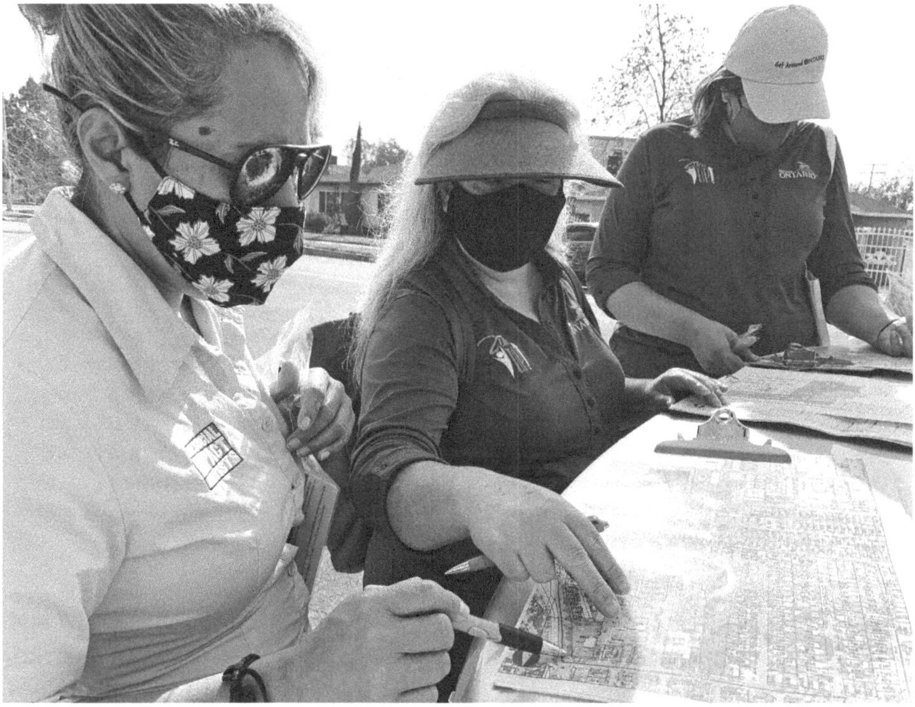

Source: Reprinted with permission of Social Impact Artists.

Figure 4-2. Social Impact Artists Community Engagement Climate Action Team

and engage individual and collective curiosity, compassion, and righteous outrage (see Figure 4-2).

If people long to be heard, can we as public health practitioners engage the people who are feeling victimized, invisible, and left out of power dynamics to craft their own story, share it, and engage others? The Centers for Disease Control and Prevention (CDC) seems to think so. In May 2020, the CDC endorsed the New England School of Public Health's free online storytelling course that introduces the science and art of storytelling as an effective communication tool in public health practice (see Box 4-1).

Because at their core human interactions are laced with self-interest, storytelling must also engage the mind, heart, and senses through culturally meaningful narrative, music,

> This process will require that we awaken community wisdom (as opposed to convincing people to take a certain position), leave behind public health jargon, find relatable language, and understand the culture and language of the communities we need to engage.

Box 4-1. Online Storytelling Course

The New England Public Health Training Center's free, online storytelling course introduces the science and art of storytelling as an effective communication tool in public health practice. This effective course is geared toward public health program managers, communication specialists, and community health workers, many of whom were and are on the front lines of the COVID-19 pandemic providing lifesaving health services and information directly in the neighborhoods where they live and serve. The training is one-hour, self-paced instruction, provides continuing education credits, and shows practitioners how to tell stories through various formats such as writing, data, and videos. It is a practical impact tool for public health workers (for more information, see: www.nephtc.org/enrol/index.php?id=129).[3]

If public health is the science of prevention, it is important to look at the ecosystems where communities are centered and the most effective structures for communicating within these ecosystems. As public health leaders, we are called to understand and empathize with the lived experiences of those we serve, the social determinants of health, and the structures and biases that have created inequity. Storytelling is a useful tool that crosses cultural boundaries and helps public health departments, leaders, and practitioners to address inequities and bias in our systems and modes of care. Storytelling also teaches us to be better listeners, helping us to move past clinical definitions and metrics of health "to the complexities of story that allow for the human aspects of illness to be absorbed and understood."[4]

song, photos, and art (see Box 4-2). Annette Simmons explains in *The Story Factor* that the concept of self-interest lies at the very center of any psychological model for influencing others.[5] Storytelling's psychological goal is to influence by connecting in some way to listeners, community members, and self-interest. Advertisers and successful social media influencers inherently understand this. This can present "kaleidoscopic targets" because as change agents public health advocates must work with conscious and subconscious interests and factors that are ever unfolding.[6]

Another proven strategy to assist with effectively engaging self- and community interest is to hold focus groups and beta test communication and storytelling materials. Testing can occur with as few as three to five community members who represent the demographics and lived experience of the population to be reached. These types of feedback loops have been invaluable in my efforts with groups working to improve community health.

Box 4-2. Community Spotlight: El Sol Neighborhood Educational Center

An impactful example of engaging the heart and mind through culturally centered storytelling that engages individual, familial, and community interests is El Sol Neighborhood Educational Center's (El Sol) COVID-19 interventions. El Sol uses comic strips and even theatrical plays created by the community to cut through cultural vaccine hesitancies—mistrust, myths, the perceived role of politics, and fears—to tell their community story of why Latinx and Black communities should vaccinate themselves and their families. Their methods focused on the intersections of the Latinx family as a target audience and incorporated the vulnerabilities and interests of parents, youth, and grandparents.

Note: Learn more about El Sol at: https://www.elsolnec.org/news-and-media/covid-19-response.

For example, in 2021, when society was experiencing the fatigue resulting from the pandemic and California stay-at-home orders, my company, Social Impact Artists (SIA), was charged with creating promotional materials for vaccine education programs to coincide with the San Bernardino County vaccination rollout (learn more about SIA at: https://www.thesocialimpactartists.com). We were working with San Antonio Regional Hospital, Loma Linda Medical Center, and the San Bernardino Department of Public Health to provide free community vaccination workshops. We worked with five San Bernardino Latina community health workers who represented the population we hoped to engage. These women cocreated and edited our engagement materials, ensuring that the language and photos would engage the self-interests of the parents and grandparents they were designed to reach. We compensated them each at a rate of $17 an hour to help us to conceive, coauthor, and review the materials. SIA also compensated them at the same rate to promote the workshops, remind participants to attend, and follow up with attendees if they had questions. Because of these efforts, the workshops were very successful (see Figure 4-3).

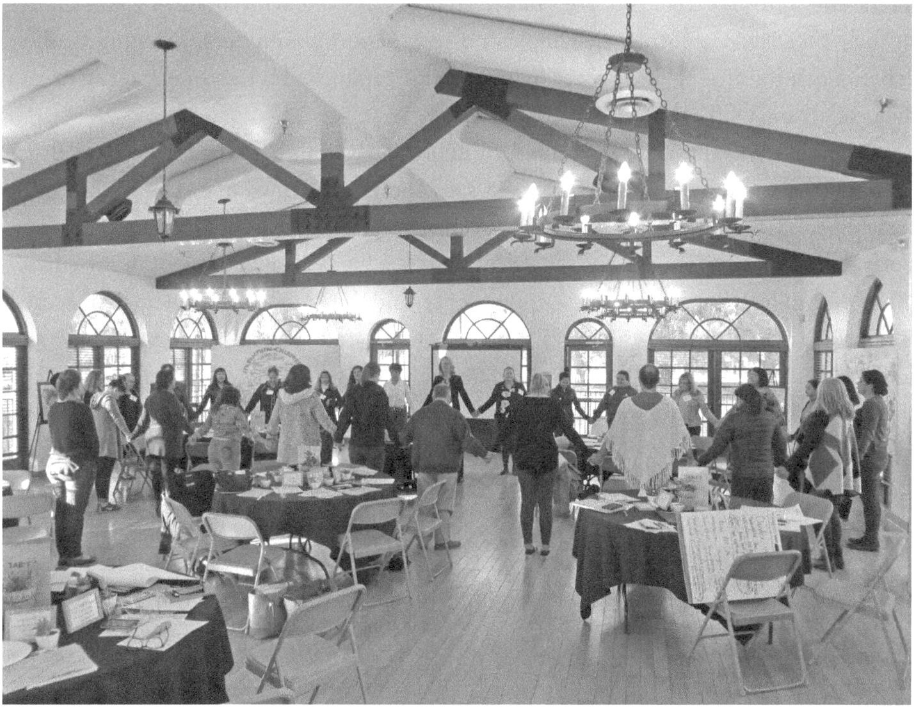

Source: Reprinted with permission of Social Impact Artists.
Photo Credit: Karen Thompson, City of Ontario Planning Department

Figure 4-3. Collective Impact Retreat

Strategies for Cross-Cultural Connections

The best stories help us to cross class, cultural, national, and gender lines and to empathize with people and situations, changing us as consumers of the story and ultimately changing the world. The best storytellers are those who live the experience they describe. Videos, poems, and novels create sparks that ignite imaginations, longings, and righteous anger, giving us the courage, motivation, and examples to change systems that no longer serve us and those who are vulnerable. The messaging bypasses our socially constructed caution and creates associations with others that speak directly to human connections, creating guardrails to guide us through the complex, frightening, messy, and heartbreaking circumstances that contribute to pandemics, disinformation, anti-science ideology, inaction, and inertia.

Most important, when we engage and listen to the community, we grow our own humility and learn how to address our implicit biases, avoiding future failures. *We become teachable.* For instance, I recall a teachable moment when I worked on my master's capstone project focused on economic mobility models for youth living below the national poverty level. I explored youth asset mapping as a viable engagement and data collection methodology to assess economic mobility. I enjoyed working with about 14 youth leaders in their Ontario, California, neighborhood teen action committees, listening to their experiences, training them in asset mapping, and exploring models of engagement and data collection.

Although my approach was rooted in appreciative inquiry, when I developed the training, the youth quickly helped me to spot some of my own biases. An admirer of certain aspects of Steve Jobs's journey as a change maker and technology entrepreneur, I quoted one of his more famous statements and used it as an anchor piece in my curriculum. The slide was met with a deafening silence, and the group of teens who had seemed so engaged when the training began looked bewildered. Jocelyn, a savvy, funny, and intelligent 17-year-old and the identified leader in the group, kindly pointed out to me that she had no idea who I was talking about and why he and his statement should matter to the group! iPhones, MacBooks, and their origin stories were my cherished construct, and Jobs's story was my emotional connection, not theirs. I leaned into the moment and asked Jocelyn and the others to share with me whom they admired and any quotes that inspired them to create visions of change. They shared with energy, and I learned a valuable lesson about visioning and storytelling that I carry into my work to this day (see Figure 4-4).

How Stories Grip and Transform

Writers create a simulation of human consciousness. For instance, to read a page in a novel "is to experience the consciousness of a character as if we were them."[7] During the 19th century, slave narratives brought white readers into the lives of American slaves

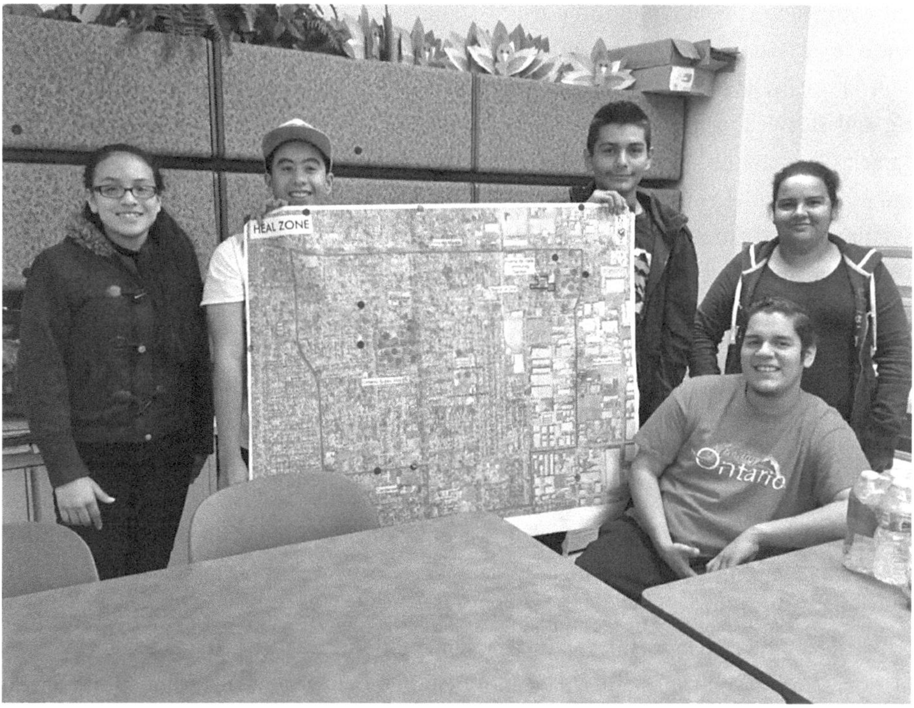

Source: Reprinted with permission of Social Impact Artists.
Photo Credit: Evette De Luca

Figure 4-4. Ontario Youth Leaders

trapped in bondage. Books such as Harriet Beecher Stowe's bestseller *Uncle Tom's Cabin* are thought to have helped bring about the American Civil War, which brought slavery to an end.[8]

During the 2021 American presidential inauguration, Amanda Gorman, the first national youth poet laureate of the United States, enthralled the Biden inauguration audience (and social media) with "The Hill We Climb," a poem she wrote after witnessing the 2021 siege on the US Capitol, which artfully referenced our painful history and instilled hope in our future: we were not broken, simply unfinished. She envisioned a way for Americans to come together, to heal, and to find our footing somewhere along a rocky path for change within "a union of purpose."

It's important to understand that good storytelling makes us human. Amanda's poem grounded us in our humanity and the humanity of others whom we may not understand. When we couple this fundamental grounding with community cocreation and social and health data, we can be confident that resulting engagement design will be effective, creating a space that residents and stakeholders own to grow collective muscle for compassion and community care. We also tap into our need for connection and self-expression (people long to be heard). There is simply no way to understand our world or set visions for change without stories.

And finally, let's look at Netflix, arguably one of America's more well-known streaming and storytelling platforms. In 2018, Netflix secured a deal with former president Barack Obama and former first lady Michelle Obama to produce documentary series and movies for their streaming service. In a statement, President Obama said, "We hope to cultivate and curate the talented, inspiring, creative voices who are able to promote greater empathy and understanding between peoples, and help them share their stories with the entire world."[9]

It is fascinating to learn from the evolution of the Obamas as storytellers, their wins, and failures. The author of multiple books collectively, President and First Lady Obama are gifted storytellers; their words and delivery fueled a movement and catapulted Barack Obama into office in 2008. Despite his gifts, we witnessed President Obama's grueling struggle to pass the Affordable Care Act (ACA), one of his most significant accomplishments, and one of our nation's most transformational public health policies (one that benefited 35 million ACA and Medicare beneficiaries who now have access to a series of preventative health care services).[10] It could be argued that his administration focused primarily on the development, rollout, implementation, and technology of the ACA legislation. What about storytelling? His administration had a powerful opportunity to tell the story of the lives that were saved and transformed as a result of the ACA, a story that we can all continue to tell. By 2016, 9 in 10 Americans had health insurance because of the ACA. My mom, my husband, and I were among these beneficiaries.

Yet the Obama administration—and many of us—missed the opportunity to connect with American hearts, through our inherent hard-wiring for stories, to cross class and cultural lines to reflect on the impact that the ACA had. We failed to effectively shape and thus control the narrative. As a beneficiary and public health change agent, I also failed to contribute my voice and experience to this collective narrative.

The Obamas' move to Netflix demonstrates lessons learned from this experience. Consider their 2022 streaming documentary *Our Great National Parks*, where the former president serves as host and narrator, tackling important issues such as climate action, scientific research, and wildlife conservation. The ACA taught us all critical lessons: as host, he meets us where we live (on our couch, remote in hand), lets the animals and breathtaking landscape tell the story, and invites us to empathize and see things differently, engaging our senses and hearts first, thus capturing our attention to consider commitment and action. As viewers, we are brought into the story, invited to experience nature alongside him, and guided through a process of discovery that encourages us to be curious, connected, and engaged.

The words of former first lady Michelle Obama offer an important pivot as change agents from government to storytelling: "Barack and I have always believed in the power of storytelling to inspire us, to make us think differently about the world around us, and to help us open our minds and hearts to others."[11] Theirs is an interesting journey of failures incorporating nimbleness and scaled communication platforms for public health leaders to learn. As community organizers, attorneys, president and first lady, and authors, they have used storytelling as a fulcrum for their work.

In other words, authentic community engagement creates deeper connections and meaningful spaces to address health and social inequity and drive positive transformation. Effective storytelling throughout a movement's life cycle can catalyze change in exponential ways, get the right people involved, illustrate meaningful impact, *and* carve energized spaces for community and stakeholders to be vulnerable, share openly, and continue to lead in transformative ways. Effective storytelling also motivates and imparts the courage and stamina needed to change imperfect systems, address heartbreaking inequity, and rewire faulty systems. And this is, at its core, the challenge and opportunity for public health leaders.

Those Who Are Closest Need to Develop the Vision

It is not down on any map; true places never are.

–Herman Melville[12]

One of the best ways to ensure that organization and initiatives "stay the course" is for people and movements to remember the stories they cocreate or are told. If we generate no stories, our followers will be left to chart their own paths without guidance.[13] Communication must happen again and again, a perpetual ground hog's day of dialogue, except that we are able to modify and improve as we move along. This ongoing need for clarity is not as difficult as it may sound, especially if we adopt a communal, populist approach: a community engagement and storytelling loop that begins with logic models at the forefront and is peppered and fueled by impact stories throughout.[14] Impact stories live on a spectrum that can include 30–60-second Instagram reels or stories, 2.5–4-minute scripted videos, and 5–10-minute TikTok videos. Community members can take the lead in these, augmenting the reach and capacity of public health departments and community-based organizations. And many of the people that we need to reach, in rural communities, disenfranchised communities, and ethnic enclaves, will more readily consume the stories generated by their friends, neighbors, and peers.

Stories Animate Questions. Communities Create the Answers.

A successful story distills our world into something that we feel we can digest and understand. It is crucial to analyze complex social issues and design health strategies using storytelling methods: film, graphics, popular education, and narrative stories. These methods help us to move beyond data points to connect with the story behind the data so that people can define *and* find themselves and their self-interest within or connected

> We live in a time where facts even seem subordinate to stories. Providing "reasons why" through storytelling allows the audience to understand context and experience emotion and thereby activates shifts that can lead to transformation. This is because stories are contagious.

to an issue. Simply sharing facts does not connect audiences to community members' sides regarding various issues, whether racism, health equity, inequity, the environment, or something else.

Religions successfully use stories to engage members and, ideally, to negotiate daily life with compassion and wisdom. Parents use family stories to create a sense of connection and understanding in our children. Community-based organizations use popular stories and popular education to build understanding and action. The concept of popular education as a methodology came from a Brazilian educator and writer, Paulo Freire, who was interested in literacy education for poor and politically disempowered people in his country. This is different from formal education in that it is inclusive, is accessible, and addresses the issues people face in their own communities. It aims to empower people who feel socially and politically marginalized to lead their own learning and to effect social change.[15]

Rejecting the "empty vessel" approach to education, popular education develops grassroots leaders who can be powerful allies in engagement and storytelling, helping to give voice to cultures that may feel silenced. An excellent example of this is a partner organization that my team and I enjoy working with, El Sol Neighborhood Educational Center, which I referenced earlier. El Sol created *CHW Comics*, a play and comic book story featuring culturally relevant educational resources to help people of all ages understand COVID-19 and community solutions in an appealing format (see Figure 4-5, Vacunas vs COVID-19). The comics cover vaccination and mental health topics related to the virus and encourage community members to obtain accurate information from trusted sources in the hope of combating misinformation and disinformation.

In short, popular education is a collective effort in which a high degree of participation is expected from everybody. Teachers and learners aren't two distinct groups; rather, everyone teaches and everyone learns! If we ground our engagement and storytelling in the truths embraced by popular education, we may also be able to learn from and ultimately overcome power struggles to enervate our work.

Effective Community Engagement and Storytelling Assets

It's people, not plot, that we are most interested in. "It's the plight of specific, flawed and fascinating individuals that makes us cheer, weep and ram our heads into the sofa cushion."[16] So put the people to work. In engagement and storytelling, community members

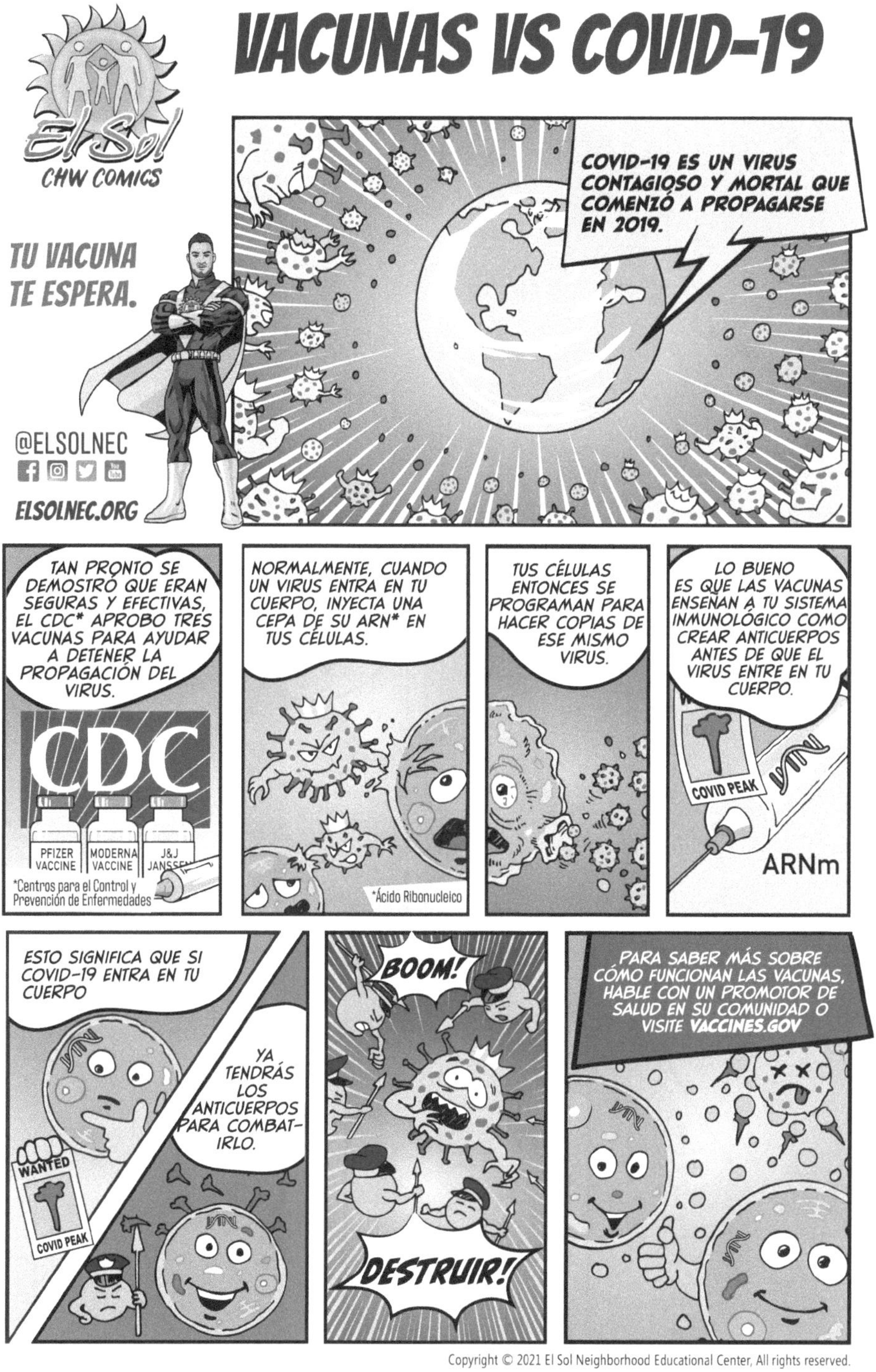
VACUNAS VS COVID-19
El Sol
CHW COMICS
TU VACUNA TE ESPERA.
@ELSOLNEC
ELSOLNEC.ORG
COVID-19 ES UN VIRUS CONTAGIOSO Y MORTAL QUE COMENZÓ A PROPAGARSE EN 2019.
TAN PRONTO SE DEMOSTRÓ QUE ERAN SEGURAS Y EFECTIVAS, EL CDC* APROBO TRES VACUNAS PARA AYUDAR A DETENER LA PROPAGACIÓN DEL VIRUS.
CDC
PFIZER VACCINE
MODERNA VACCINE
J&J
*Centros para el Control y Prevención de Enfermedades
NORMALMENTE, CUANDO UN VIRUS ENTRA EN TU CUERPO, INYECTA UNA CEPA DE SU ARN* EN TUS CÉLULAS.
*Ácido Ribonucleico
TUS CÉLULAS ENTONCES SE PROGRAMAN PARA HACER COPIAS DE ESE MISMO VIRUS.
LO BUENO ES QUE LAS VACUNAS ENSEÑAN A TU SISTEMA INMUNOLÓGICO COMO CREAR ANTICUERPOS ANTES DE QUE EL VIRUS ENTRE EN TU CUERPO.
COVID PEAK
ARNm
ESTO SIGNIFICA QUE SI COVID-19 ENTRA EN TU CUERPO
WANTED
COVID PEAK
YA TENDRÁS LOS ANTICUERPOS PARA COMBAT-IRLO.
BOOM!
DESTRUIR!
PARA SABER MÁS SOBRE CÓMO FUNCIONAN LAS VACUNAS, HABLE CON UN PROMOTOR DE SALUD EN SU COMUNIDAD O VISITE VACCINES.GOV
Copyright © 2021 El Sol Neighborhood Educational Center, All rights reserved.

Source: Reprinted with permission of El Sol (https://www.elsolnec.org/news-and-media/covid-19-response).

Figure 4-5. Vacunas vs COVID-19

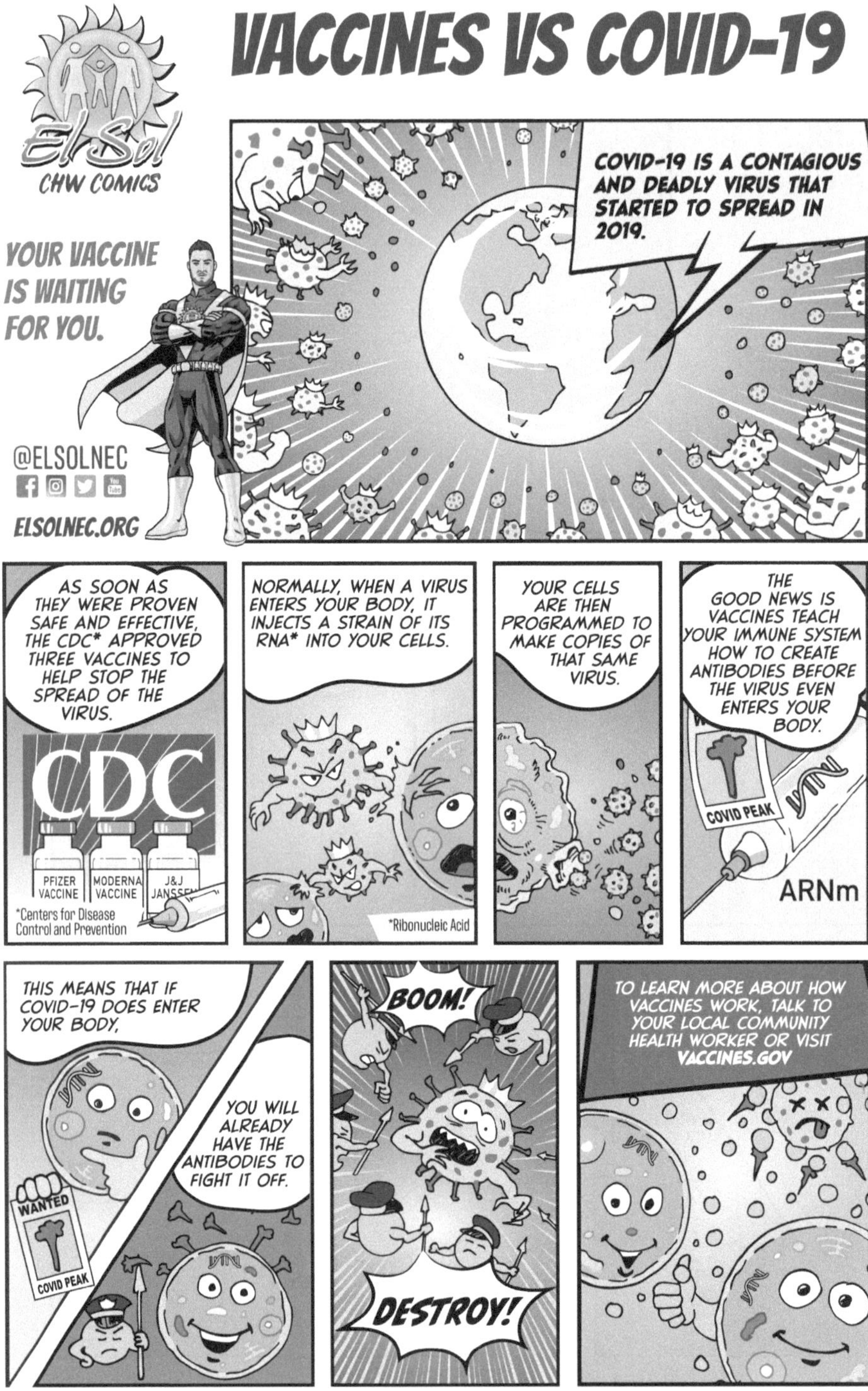

Figure 4-5. (Continued)

are our greatest—and most sustainable—asset. Engagement and the stories that fuel it become more sustainable and go viral when *they* lead. When community members design and tell their own narratives providing extra little details that load the story with emotion, they can and will activate people to learn and change. This leadership can take many forms: consider having community members facilitate or co-facilitate public health meetings. An example of this is how my company, SIA, trained four Inland Empire residents to lead Community Health Improvement Association meetings in the City of Ontario and to lead regional focus groups to assess public health and equity needs across Inland Empire in California. These residents, most of whom were Latinx immigrants, understood their environment, their neighbors, and their vision for their communities far better than the city planners and public health practitioners whom we worked with ever could.

Rooted in their neighborhoods for decades, these SIA-trained Inland Empire residents understand the people who live around them because they walk side by side with them, take the bus with them, share meals, shop with them, party with them, and attend church with them. Many are already arbiters of engagement and conflict resolvers. These women also know how to tell a story to engage community members, how to cut through the dynamics of mistrust and misinformation by sharing their *own* stories, and how to engage their neighbors in a vision for the future that includes their voices and desires.

At the onset, communities may need to exercise courage, and this can be cultivated and fostered through specific types of support. Training, investment in equipment and technology, mentoring, and practicing facilitation—these all can manifest more effective engagement and storytelling.

Best Practices

Best practices include everything from developing vision stories to creating photographic records and videos as well as engaging in journalistic activities.

Vision Stories

Public health leaders can turn to those who are closest to the issues to codevelop vision stories. Visioning stories can be journeys where we "walk side by side" to create new, impactful solutions, creating a vision for a world within which we can all find better versions of ourselves. An impactful vision story connects with people, imparting energy that shrinks immediate frustrations "in light of the promise of tomorrow."[17]

These stories can be especially helpful when working through complexity and systems change. For example, through video storytelling on its website landing page, Change Elemental shows a viewer the people within its organization who are leading multisectoral racial equity strategies in Washington, DC (for more information, see: www.changeelemental.org). Their mandate is to drive systems change, yet they focus on love, dignity, justice, and fun—with storytelling as an anchor for the multiple organizations working through extreme complexity. Sounds like a complicated stew: systems change, love, dignity, justice, and fun—how can you describe this? At under 2:20 minutes, their vision story shows you the people leading the work and describes a vision that feels like a narrative truth and connects with the urgency of the moment.

Photovoice

Photovoice is a form of community-based participatory research created by C. Wang and M. A. Burris in 1997 (for more on their research, see: https://pubmed.ncbi.nlm.nih.gov/9158980). This type of research incorporates resident-level points of view. Grounded in reciprocity and social action, it is a process by which communities can identify, represent, and enhance their neighborhoods by using specific photographic techniques (for more information, see: https://globalhealth.duke.edu/news/what-photovoice). It uses photographs as a tool to identify issues and solutions. For example, in my work with Ontario Healthy Eating, Active Living Zone, we worked with the Ontario Planning Department, Kaiser Permanente, and community partners to train resident leaders in the Photovoice framework to identify issues related to poor walkability and their perceptions of traffic impact in their neighborhoods.

After being trained to use cameras and to understand the Photovoice framework and our process, residents walked their neighborhoods with family and friends to take pictures to answer the question, Are your neighborhoods safe to walk and bike? Residents then took pictures to answer the question from their point of view. For example, one woman took pictures of a particular street in her neighborhood that lacked sidewalks yet had high patterns of foot traffic. Another took photos of street intersections where many automobile-pedestrian accidents had occurred as a result of high automobile traffic volume and speeding.

The Ontario Planning Department collected and printed the photos, and the residents analyzed and ranked those that best represented the issues in their neighborhood. We also documented what the residents said as they discussed their perspectives and priorities. Residents offered the Ontario Planning Department solutions that would improve walkability; the department then incorporated some of these solutions to create safer pedestrian infrastructure in the Ontario HEAL Zone, including adding sidewalks. The photos and documented quotes from the resident leaders would become elemental components of our visual storytelling, including reports, websites, social media, and marketing materials. These were their stories, their photos, reflecting their neighborhoods, their hopes, and their solutions.

Community Participatory Video

Participatory video is a form of scriptless community storytelling in which a group of people create their own film. The idea behind this technique is that making a short video is accessible and relatively easy, especially because videos can be filmed and edited using smartphones and social media apps. The growing affordability of and access to digital video technologies have led to a steady increase in the use of participatory video as a research methodology.[18] Much like Photovoice, participatory video is also an effective and fun way to bring the community together to analyze and create solutions to community problems, elevating their interests, perspectives, and solutions. Communities can control their narrative, explore their power, and bring challenges and solutions across communities and forward to decision makers. It is also a highly useful tool to engage and mobilize marginalized communities. Completed films can be used to promote awareness and foster learning across communities within target audiences. Framework components include training, filming, and editing activities and final dissemination of the film. Insightshare offers toolkits, methodology, and key project videos to further explore this technique and its potential impact (for more information, see: https://insightshare.org).

Citizen Journalism

Citizen journalism involves content produced by private citizens who are not journalists and who disseminate information through social media, websites, and the internet. It creates avenues for private citizens to actively collect and distribute information and stories. With the efficiency of readily available technology, citizens can often report events and information faster than traditional media outlets. This technique is not without controversy, for lacking a formal framework, it can be subjective and heavily opinionated.[19] Yet it also provides avenues for residents to detail their or others' lived experiences while bypassing the power dynamics that exist with traditional media outlets and their control of community narratives. Of particular interest, and perhaps opportunity, is whether information from a unofficial source may enhance the credibility of official government health messages.

One of the most courageous and important examples of citizen journalism occurred when Darnella Frazier, age 17, filmed the police misconduct that resulted in the murder of 46-year-old George Floyd in May 2020. She filmed Officer Derek Chavin's knee on Mr. Floyd's neck for more than nine excruciating minutes. Frazier's brave actions and her sharing of her footage on social media provided evidence of the violence and structural racism in play on American streets that traditional media outlets could and potentially would not have captured or shared. Her footage activated a worldwide swell of support for the Black Lives Matter movement and highlighted "the crucial role of citizens in journalists' quests for truth and justice," resulting in a Pulitzer special citation and award.[20]

Citizen health journalism is a young and not fully explored concept that couples citizen journalism with community health workers. An interesting example is Vivo Rio, an organization that trains community health workers to employ the philosophy and technique of citizen journalism to offer unique insights about the health of their own communities.[21] Sacrificing their own safety, Chinese citizen journalists were instrumental in shining a light on the true impact of COVID-19 in Wuhan during the early days of the emerging pandemic. Their videos documented a reality that was not represented in traditional government media outlets and were widely shared on social media, galvanizing international action.

Storytelling is an increasingly valuable tool for public health practitioners to use when communicating health information to the public because of its ability to punch with emotion, thereby creating connection and comprehension. Public health leaders have opportunities to engage community and culture bearers to author and coauthor critical health messaging in innovative and meaningful ways. In this era of complexity, it is imperative that we turn to the power of story, engage and center the people who live the story to author it, and cocreate a network of human consciousness, a sense of control, wonder, and ultimately a sense of hope.

So let us leave behind a country
better than the one we were left with…
our people diverse and beautiful will emerge,
battered and beautiful.

–Amanda Gorman, *The Hill We Climb*[22]

REFERENCES

1. Community Wealth Partners. Engaging stakeholders in developing strategies: a field guide. Available at: https://communitywealth.com/wp-content/uploads/2020/06/Stakeholder-Engagement-Field-Guide.pdf. Accessed August 31 2022.
2. Monks E. The glow and the shadow of the halo effect of influencers. CRISP. October 28, 2020. Accessible at: https://www.crispthinking.com/blog/halo-effect-of-influencers. Accessed August 31, 2022.
3. New England Public Health Training Center. Storytelling for public health. Available at: www.nephtc.org/enrol/index.php?id=129. Accessed August 27, 2022.
4. Pallaj EL, Tran K. Narrative health: using story to explore definitions of health and address bias in health care. *The Permanente J.* 2019;23(1):1.
5. Simmons A. *The Story Factor: Secrets of Influence from the Art of Story Telling.* 1st ed. New York, NY: Basic Books; 2001:66.
6. Simmons A. *The Story Factor: Secrets of Influence from the Art of Story Telling.* 1st ed. New York, NY: Basic Books; 2001:107.

7. Storr W. *Science of Storytelling: Why Stories Make Us Human and How to Tell Them Better.* 2nd ed. London, UK: William Collins; 2020:208.
8. Storr W. *Science of Storytelling: Why Stories Make Us Human and How to Tell Them Better.* 2nd ed. London, UK: William Collins; 2020:208.
9. Holloway D. Barack and Michelle Obama sign Netflix production deal. Variety.com. May 21, 2018. Accessible at: https://variety.com/2018/digital/news/barack-michelle-obama-netflix-deal-1202817723. Accessed August 29, 2022.
10. HHS Press Office. New reports show record 35 million people enrolled in coverage related to the Affordable Care Act, with historic 21 million people enrolled in Medicaid expansion coverage. HHS.gov. April 29, 2022. https://www.hhs.gov/about/news/2022/04/29/new-reports-show-record-35-million-people-enrolled-in-coverage-related-to-the-affordable-care-act.html. Accessed August 29, 2022.
11. Holloway D. Barack and Michelle Obama sign Netflix production deal. Variety.com. May 21, 2018. Accessible at: https://variety.com/2018/digital/news/barack-michelle-obama-netflix-deal-1202817723. Accessed August 29, 2022.
12. Melville, H. *Moby-Dick or, The Whale.* Penguin Group; 1988: 61.
13. Simmons A. *The Story Factor: Secrets of Influence from the Art of Story Telling.* 1st ed. New York, NY: Basic Books; 2001:66.
14. Valerio L. Community-led change: how the Wells Fargo Regional Foundation builds the capacity of nonprofits and communities to shape neighborhoods together. November 28, 2018. Accessible at: https://learningforfunders.candid.org/content/case-studies/community-led-change. Accessed August 29, 2022.
15. Popednews. What is popular education? November 2005. Accessible at: http://base.socioeco.org/docs/what_is_popular_education.pdf. Accessed August 29, 2022.
16. Storr W. *Science of Storytelling: Why Stories Make Us Human and How to Tell Them Better.* 2nd ed. London, UK: William Collins; 2020:6.
17. Simmons A. *The Story Factor: Secrets of Influence from the Art of Story Telling.* 1st ed. New York, NY: Basic Books; 2001:13.
18. Marzi S. Participatory video from a distance: co-producing knowledge during the COVID-19 pandemic using smartphones. *Qual Res.* August 20, 2021. doi:10.1177/14687941211038171.
19. Min S-J. Conversation through journalism: searching for organizing principles of public and citizen journalism. *Journalism.* 2016;17(5):567–582. doi:10.1177/1464884915571298.
20. The Pulitzer Prizes. Special citations and awards. Accessible at: https://www.pulitzer.org/prize-winners-by-category/260. Accessed August 29, 2022.
21. Davis S. Citizen health journalism. *Journalism Pract.* 2017;11(2–3):319–335. doi:10.1080/17512786.2016.1230022.
22. Gorman A. *The Hill We Climb: An Inaugural Poem for the Country.* New York: Penguin; 2021.

5

Community Engagement in Action

Lisa Beczkiewicz, Sarah Garber, MS, Patrick J. Cusick, MSPH, REHS, Kim Foreman, Jennifer Muggeo, MPH, and Ana P. Novais

MISSOULA, MONTANA

Lisa Beczkiewicz and Sarah Garber, MS

In 2016, the City of Missoula was selected by the Reinvestment Fund and the Robert Wood Johnson Foundation to take part in the new Invest Health initiative. Invest Health's aim is to transform how leaders from midsize American cities work together to help low-income communities thrive, with specific attention to community features that drive health such as access to safe and affordable housing, places to play and exercise, and quality jobs.

By establishing Missoula's Invest Health team, we were able to create new ways to link community development, public health, and community engagement. We educated our city-county government and community partners on the health disparities in Missoula. They were eager to learn more on how to support resident-driven transformative change to improve health outcomes for all. In 2019, Missoula City-County Health Department leaders knew that we needed to be doing more work to engage community residents. There was an internal vision and passion for this work that aligned with national Public Health Accreditation Board standards.

The vision is to build Missoula City-County Health Equity capacity to coordinate and support civic sector leadership and city-county government officials to improve the health and wellness of all people regardless of social position or other socially determined factors such as race, ethnicity, language, disability, sexual orientation, gender, immigration status, or socioeconomic status and to build internal and external capacity to address root causes of health inequities through planning, implementations, and evaluations processes.

To accomplish this vision, a coordinator for health equity position was created and funded by Invest Health and other foundations. The coordinator for health equity partnered with a broad-based community-organizing effort to empower diverse groups to become involved in developing unique, culturally appropriate, and sustainable solutions to inequity that affect their health outcomes and well-being.

Missoula City-County Health Department has engaged in community organizing because it is a technique that addresses inequity by creating a racially and socially diverse network of everyday citizen leaders whose mission is to address local challenges affecting health, challenges such as health care access, income inequality, lack of affordable housing, and structural racism. At the root of community organizing is the goal to build relationships with and empower neighbors and everyday citizens. It is important that these individuals identify and prioritize the health inequities they are facing and be involved in creating solutions that shape our community and create systemic change to address the social determinants of health.

Also important to us is that the community organizing be led by the people most directly affected by the issues. They are the experts in their own lives and should be involved in the decisions that affect their own health and well-being. Defined as "the process by which community groups are helped to identify common problems or change targets, mobilize resources and develop and implement strategies to reach their collective goals,"[1] community organizing is about supporting community members as they build community and power together; it is about allowing them to feel seen, valued, heard, and involved in decisions that affect their health and well-being. We want to partner with our community and work to understand and address the root causes of the issues, not just the symptoms.

As a result, we have committed to community organizing as one of our community engagement approaches. As a department, we have started this effort in one of Missoula's three Invest Health neighborhoods. Most exciting for us is that another Invest Health neighborhood has also started community organizing with the support of a nonprofit in the community.

As stated earlier, we are supporting and guiding one of our Invest Health neighborhoods in building their organizing core team. The neighborhood group has built teams to take on service activities to help neighbors with individual needs; the teams advocate as a group to city council for other neighborhood needs and are developing their organizing teams so that they can build power together and have a greater impact on health disparities. To date, they have completed murals in their neighborhood, built planters around traffic circles, and installed murals at traffic circles. As well, they are currently working on a native plant garden that includes education information for residents to enjoy and care for.

This neighborhood organizing team is also entering a time of listening and engaging with the residents of the neighborhood. This involves one-on-one and group conversations that offer a space for people to share the pressures they and their families are facing and the hopes for their neighborhood, community, and future. Building relationships and trust is so important, for it enables folks to be heard, to be connected, and to find mutual common ground so that they can begin to build power together. They feel connected to something larger than themselves and together can move toward the change they envision.

> Listening is the first step, but it only goes so far. The important changes that need to happen require collective action.

At the core of this listening is meeting people where they are, holding space for feelings and reactions, and forming connections and engaging with others. Also, when we share our stories, we can connect with each other through shared experiences and our hopes for the future. This way of connecting enables us to build a strong community and is how we build authentic, engaged relationships and empower others. It is the first step in making change.

After this period of listening, the group members decide what issues they would like to focus on and which to take action on. This happens in September in each member organization and takes place within a larger, broad-based community-organizing group.

Once this discernment takes place, we move into researching the selected issue and deciding where, when, and how to act on it together. This may involve meeting and working with city and/or county staff or consultants on rezoning policies, for example, or attending planning meetings and city council meetings. It may require meeting with county commissioners, attending board of health meetings, and more. This is where we can take any version of a complicated civic issue, demystify it, develop solutions, and implement new policies, services, or programs.

Focusing on policy change is important, but it needs to involve community voices, and we need to support power building within our community. It is vitally important that our community members be able to build power with each other rather than having us hold power over our community. They must take on the social determinants of health in the "world as it is" and move health and wellness forward to get us to the "world as it should be." They determine the work we do.

Both the Missoula City-County Health Department and the neighborhood organization we are working with are members of a broad-based community-organizing group called Common Good Missoula. Common Good Missoula comprises 35 community-organizing members who come together to work on issues that affect the entire community. Members have greater influence and impact working as a group rather than as individuals. The community groups that are members of Common Good Missoula have just that, and this influence and impact also allows us to build relationships of trust across racial, faith, economic, and geographic lines. Common Good Missoula's member organizations include All Nations Health Center (Missoula's Urban Indian Health Center), labor unions, faith communities, neighborhoods, and other nonprofits.

Missoula City-County Health Department also partners with other Common Good Missoula community organizers to provide free community-organizing training to individuals throughout the community, including leaders in Invest Health neighborhoods. Indigenous and Native leaders in the community have also provided a workshop to more than 200 non-Indigenous Missoulians called Wrestling with the Truth of Colonization that has helped participants acknowledge their role in colonization and face the true history of the Missoula Valley. The purpose of this training is to move Common Good Missoula and its member organizations toward being "a true interracial organization built of trust and allyship."

As noted, the fundamental method of this broad-based community organizing is to build relationships in the public arena that are authentic and caring. Our focus is on this relational community building because, at the core, it connects people through their motivations to protect and restore their own well-being and that of their families and their community. We focus on this broad base of support because without it health inequities will persist and the needed change to social determinants of health for those most affected will not happen.

Common Good Missoula and its member organizations, including Missoula City-County Health Department, worked together during COVID-19 to support the organizing of tech-charging stations to offer internet access to people applying for government aid during business closures. Common Good Missoula also supported the opening of a pantry of essential nonfood items for community members. As well, partner organizations worked to support the formation of the housing trust fund, the landlord liaison position, and a citizen's oversight committee at the City of Missoula. During this time, multiple citizens' academies on housing and workers' rights were held on Zoom, and these functions were attended by more than 500 people. In addition to all this, one Missoula County neighborhood and two City of Missoula neighborhoods were supported in shaping neighborhood development and community building.

The entire membership also came together in May 2022 at a community event called a Founding Celebration. This event celebrated the work that has been done and allowed the member organizations "to publicly commit to continuing to engage their members, our neighbors, and each other" to create a more equitable Missoula for all. At roll call, 418 people were in attendance, with more arriving throughout the evening, among them community members, city and county staff, and state, county, and city elected officials.

As we continue this journey, our health department is still exploring other ways to include community members in our community organizing. We are exploring how to do this as we implement our strategies to affect social determinants of health, all while continuing to provide service and advocacy for our community. As we continue to support our Invest Health neighborhoods and organizations within Common Good Missoula, how can we go even further and incorporate community organizing into more of the work we do? We envision some ways to do this, which include working with our community health workers, our home-visiting program, and our immunization clinic to find clients, patients, and other community members who are interested in becoming involved in community organizing. The goal is to enable folks who have lived experience to have a say in policy and program changes. To realize this vision, various health department staff attended training in July 2022 provided by Common Good Missoula and its sister organization in Spokane, Washington, called Organizing for Health Equity. The training focused on community organizing in health care, clinics, and public health.

So, the work continues. We are committed to building more relationships and developing deep trust as we come together to discern the issues the teams would like to tackle, support their information-gathering and research activities, and support the community members and community organizations we work with as they act to make meaningful changes to reduce health inequities in our community. We are excited to build the world we *all* need through innovative and meaningful engagement and shared decision-making with members of our community.

CLEVELAND, OHIO

Patrick J. Cusick, MSPH, REHS, and Kim Foreman

Defining community engagement is tricky because traditionally, agencies start defining, designing, and approaching community engagement from an external and somewhat siloed space, often removed from the actual community intended to be served. Going forward, our learned experience informs us that we should instead ask how communities would like to be involved or participate, allowing them to define the best way to engage.

As a community of health practitioners, advocates, and leaders, we must ask ourselves what the end goal of engagement is. Are we just working from a transactional or programmatic definition of engagement, checking the box? Or are we working on partnering and cultivating an inclusive experience, with the end goal of sustaining the authenticity of the engagement, relationships, and real systems change?

As the Cleveland Healthy Home Data Collaborative demonstrated, it was necessary to expand our understanding of the concept and adjust our processes in a continuous fashion throughout the program. Community engagement became an integral portion of not only problem identification but also solution creation as we strived to ensure equitable outcomes. It is at this intersection of the two distinct issues—community engagement as a stand-alone concept as well as a process—that we as public health practitioners can bring into sharper focus a broader understanding and integration of community engagement. By doing so, we will be better positioned to improve community health outcomes.

A local effort that has community members involved at every stage needs to become the standard for equity and accessibility going forward. The intentional incorporation of

Box 5-1. Community Engagement as a Process

Community engagement as a process must be understood to be a repeating cycle following the framework titled "10 Essential Public Health Services" as outlined by the Centers for Disease Control and Prevention (see Figure 5-1, The 10 Essential Public Health Services). This cycle flows from assessment, through policy development (or improvement), through to assurance. This repeating cycle strives to center the activities within public health agencies and partner organizations on a health equity-based framework.

Note: To learn more about "10 Essential Public Health Services," visit https://www.cdc.gov/publichealthgateway/publichealthservices/essentialhealthservices.html.

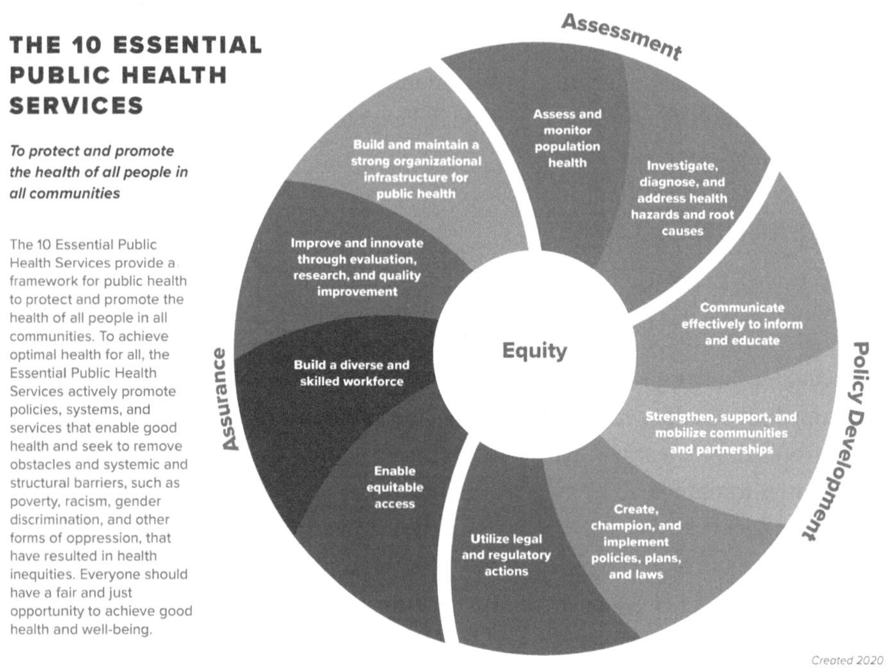

Source: Reprinted from Centers for Disease Control and Prevention.[2]

Figure 5-1. The 10 Essential Public Health Services

community concerns into existing public health strategies and programs is integral to ensuring that the evolving needs of the public are central to the efforts of the agencies and organizations tasked with serving those same communities (see Box 5-1).

The Collaborative Takes Shape

The Cleveland Healthy Home Data Collaborative began in June 2015 with the express goal of examining and addressing environmental health issues in residential units, specifically asthma triggers and lead poisoning exposures. The collaborative was designed with Environmental Health Watch, a community organization focused on environmental justice and community engagement as the lead agency, in partnership with the Cleveland Department of Public Health and MetroHealth System (known locally as MetroHealth). The collaborative believed in promoting regenerative environments and communities by supporting the continuous enhancement of health, justice, and prosperity while maintaining respect for the natural, social, cultural, and historical value of place. Together, with funding and support from The BUILD Health Challenge (BUILD), the team sought to help reduce the future incidence of asthma-related emergency room visits or other health encounters.

At the heart of the work was the community need, continually expressed, of remedying substandard housing. The problem was rampant in the urban core of Cleveland. Compounding the issue was the lack of transparency for renters about the health and safety issues in the rental stock available even though local regulatory efforts to inspect housing for code violations and lead poisoning cases resulted in residential unit inspections. The siloed approach to asthma and lead poisoning programs and the rental property complaint inspections processes in place were both ineffective for residents' needs at the time—artifacts of the regulations and programs in the local and state codified ordinances, administrative codes, and civic organization structures.

The medical community was also concerned about both asthma triggers and lead exposures from the residences where children lived or spent significant amounts of time. Health care concerns were frequently centered on office interactions and hospitalization issues; but once children's acute medical needs were met, they were returned to unsafe residences, which resulted in further exposures and exacerbations for asthma and lead poisoning.

Initial assessments of these core issues and conversations with community members revealed that while public records of violations and lead investigations existed, the process for accessing, reviewing, and collating issues between programs proved cumbersome. Some information was electronic, some was on paper records, and all access was initially routed through public information request processes. Community members seeking the information were dissuaded by the outdated process. There was also an assessment of the existing programs, policies, regulations, and inspection and enforcement of the related issues; however, the assessment was not accomplishing the intended outcomes: safer housing, fewer cases of lead poisoning, and more effective regulatory efforts.

A Framework for Change

In an effort to address these challenges, the collaborative sought to develop, first, a policy agenda to push for enforcement of the existing rental registry and systematic proactive housing inspections and, second, coordination of existing silos of data in various organizations to potentially provide information directly to the public so that someone seeking to determine if a housing unit had a history of health or building violations prior to renting or buying the residence could do so easily and quickly.

Given the shared knowledge of the community's health concerns surrounding asthma and lead poisoning, the initial scope of the project was grounded in the core principles of the BUILD framework that aim to advance health and health equity: **B**old, **U**pstream, **I**ntegrated, **L**ocal, and **D**ata-driven.

- The **Bold**—or systems change—aspect of the project was designed to change severely entrenched historical separations of interests and responsibilities between city departments, health care agencies, and advocacy groups by putting them all on the same team with shared goals. Continually centering the discussions on the health outcomes with and for the community was helpful throughout the process. This ongoing centering of the community's interests as the focus of the project was core to the concept of community engagement and required the team to prioritize community views.
- **Upstream** is a more challenging target for any community engagement project, as the agencies involved may have to change deeply ingrained practices and processes within the realm of bureaucratic organizations with decades of procedures and funding challenges. It is therefore critical to ensure key leadership's buy-in. Systems change and policy change in this project required community, legislative, and administrative support and changes at the highest levels.
- **Integration** of interests, efforts, and processes was necessary both for success and to ensure that various cross-sector agencies and community members would be able to sustain the goals of the project once grant funding was consumed. Lasting change and improved outcomes required the organizational programs and processes to be incorporated into the regulations and supported by existing revenue streams, as well as to clearly demonstrate substantive impacts. While this project started with agencies that had a previous history of collaboration, these same principles supported by a community engagement process can be successful—even with new, but dedicated, partners.
- **Local** for the team meant collaborating with community members at every stage. This project began with a set of questions for focus groups that consisted of local renters and stakeholders in an effort to find existing information on residential units. Community members frequently expressed a desire to remain in the same neighborhood so that they could maintain their community connections (e.g., schools, family and friends, places of worship, and familiar environments), which informed the program's goals and strategies. By regularly collaborating with community members, the team was able to evolve the program's strategies in real time to meet the community's needs and be more effective.
- **Data-driven** approaches allowed the team to assist in identifying safer housing units, as well as to make that data directly accessible to the public. An existing city record

system was used to develop an initial webpage portal where the public could seek out information on a specific address. This initially included only building violations, but not lead hazards. These local inspection records and the existing public-facing electronic data were utilized as the starting point for making information available to the community in the ways that made sense for them.

Discussions with community members, as highlighted across the BUILD framework, ultimately shaped the collaborative's projects and its definition of community engagement. This helped foster a more meaningful form of engagement with community members to the point where the collaborative was able to weave community voices and advocacy efforts into its strategies more fully and successfully.

Engagement at Work

This project began with an initial focus on reducing asthma and lead poisoning recurrences attributable to substandard housing. Thanks to a synergy between the right partners being engaged, the community voices being validly heard, included, and incorporated into the outcomes, and a confluence of external events (including significant national and local attention to lead poisoning in the media and collective consciousness in the community), the Cleveland Healthy Home Data Collaborative was able to leverage regulatory changes to local code enforcement, with tax revenue increased to support public health and city building rental code enforcement. Further, the collaborative's efforts broadened integration of medical providers in the entire region by maintaining their awareness of the prevention and reduction of negative health outcomes from substandard housing.

It should be noted that time and alignment of public concern will always be a factor in public health. This set of data and community engagement projects began just before the Flint water crisis became publicly known in 2015 and adapted to the explosion of public health concern related to the local lead issues outlined in a broad series of articles called "Toxic Neglect" later the same year.[3,4] The synergy between these events, the articles, and rising public awareness assisted in leveraging historic changes to policies, procedures, and legislation at local, county, and state levels in the same period as this BUILD project was happening. True to the term, community engagement went from a concept to a process whereby existing stakeholders now had direct voice in shaping policy, legislation, and direction of ongoing conversations.

Lessons Learned

The Cleveland Healthy Home Data Collaborative's community engagement project has taught participants several important lessons, among them that representation matters and that there is no single approach to involving a community—indeed, that there are always more ways to engage.

Representation Matters

Organizations and practitioners usually find one or two people from the community who are "easy" to work with and use their singular voice to represent all, which is not authentic, not inclusive of multiple perspectives, and can misrepresent the true community voice(s). We must continue to dig to find representation even if the task and/or people challenge us, push against our own biases and/or beliefs of what benefits we think we are delivering.

Practitioners, institutions, and organizations must remain humble and available, have the willingness to learn and adjust on the basis of new information, and remember that engagement is an interactive process and that community needs change. We make assumptions that institutions, especially large institutions, and organizations have the capacity to do this work. We must approach engagement with an understanding that community can teach us, that there is value in the lived experience, that engagement is an exchange of ideas, and that we can all come out richer in the end.

No Such Thing as a Cookie-Cutter Approach

The concept of community engagement relies on the authentic incorporation of community members in shaping any project from conception through to completion if it is going to be validly engaged. Often, practitioners make the mistake of defining engagement as a meeting schedule or an occasion to provide information to members of the said community without first asking what is important to them. Practitioners must learn to value lived experience, to listen first and then craft an approach in partnership with community as an equitable strategy and model of engagement.

There Are Always More Ways to Engage

Following its initial work with BUILD, the Cleveland Healthy Home Data Collaborative went on to continue its efforts and found different ways to work with the community that would spark new ideas and opportunities. Using a process called journey mapping, the collaborative brought together multiple sessions of individuals in the community to discuss their processes of finding rental housing. Through this direct engagement, members of the community shared their stories and captured each step in their individual process of finding housing, identifying the difficult and the rewarding points in their journeys. These stories were then distilled into group consensus on points to keep and points to improve on, utilizing the journey mapping process to build on the successful data portal by creating a more user-friendly and accessible application designed with the community's input in this process.

Incorporating community repeatedly and in an ongoing, intentional manner is the spirit of the concept threaded throughout the process. Positive, progressive change comes about when the affected group of constituents is properly represented at the table.

NEW LONDON COUNTY, CONNECTICUT

Jennifer Muggeo, MPH

The Health Improvement Collaborative of Southeastern Connecticut's vision and values have always centered inclusion, social justice, and equity, but it was the centering of racism as a public health issue in our 2019 community health improvement plan that accelerated and focused our community engagement efforts. We recognized very early on that if we truly wanted to address structural racism and its impact on our community's health, we needed to increase authentic community engagement and follow the true subject matter experts—our community members.

The Health Improvement Collaborative is a multidisciplinary group of organizations and individuals committed to working together to create opportunities for health for all in the southern tier of New London County, Connecticut. In 2015, community members and colleagues from the Federally Qualified Health Centers, academia, social services, and community organizations answered the call from Ledge Light Health District, the local health department, and Lawrence + Memorial Hospital, the local community-based hospital, to serve on an ad hoc steering committee for their first comprehensive community health assessment (CHA) and community health improvement plan (CHIP). The steering committee grew in size, working through secondary data collection and analysis and report layout to prioritizing the health and structural concerns included in the 2016 CHIP.

Reticent to have the plan "sit on a shelf" for three years until the next one was produced, the group decided to stay together as the Health Improvement Collaborative of Southeastern Connecticut, adopting a vision of our region as a community health in body and mind that promotes access, health equity, social justice, inclusiveness, and opportunities for all.

Today, the collaborative is an active learning and advocacy community focused on addressing racism as a public health issue and committed to shifting the balance of power from large institutions to grassroots organizations and community members. Here's what we've learned, and try to live, about community engagement.

1. **First, do no harm.** For too long, like other health departments and—really—public health writ large, Ledge Light Health District and other partners on the Health

Improvement Collaborative sat in the space where our job was to educate and inform community members about things (we thought) they didn't know. We put information out there—on billboards, on fact sheets, in presentations—and stood firm in our place as "the subject matter experts." With the 2016 CHA, we worked to consult and involve our community members by focusing in our report on a survey and focus groups instead of health department and hospital data and by inviting community partners to help us decide on priorities to be included in the assessment plan. We thought we were on top of this community engagement stuff!

The fact is that our actions, like those of others before us, were extractive and harmful to our community members. We added to the significant disconnect between systems of care and the people they serve, we reinforced old false narratives, and we used our community members by taking their stories to make our work look good to apply for grants—all with good intentions to be sure, but these efforts had harmful impacts. They eroded what little trust our community members might have held and reinforced the idea that we were another government agency, here with bureaucratic requirements and restrictions that rendered our nice words about community engagement meaningless.

In planning the 2019 CHA and CHIP, and with feedback from community partners that we had, in fact, repeated these harmful practices, we were committed to doing better. We recognized the need to go back to community members to share the data we had collected, to make sure we had the narratives right from their perspectives, to dig deeper into the whys and hows based on their lived experiences in our community. And to be honest with them—and ourselves—about what could and could not change. So, when a group of community members joined us as "community ambassadors" to review the data from the 2019 CHA and told us that childcare expenses were a significant stressor, we had to be honest about our ability to create change in that space. We *were* able to work with them to address another concern they raised regarding how people are treated when accessing local food pantries. These discussions led to the development of our Food to People Program and the creation of our Food Justice Action Team.

2. **Step back and let the experts work.** "Oh, we're going to do community engagement now, here we go!" We had funding, we had a job description and posting, but we had no candidates. Thank goodness. We realized that there were many community groups and individuals already doing incredible community engagement work, so there was no need for the collaborative or health department to create a "community engagement specialist" position and reinvent the wheel. We worked with our funder to reallocate those salary dollars and subcontract with community-based organizations. Our partnership grants were intentionally and specifically designed to have as little paperwork/application/reporting burden as possible and to support existing community engagement work.

We were not investing in building their capacity; we were instead sharing our resources so that they might be able to invest in building ours. They've been graciously sharing their insights and guidance with the institutional partners on the Health Improvement Collaborative and in doing so building connections between the community members they are already engaged with and the collaborative.

Another group of experts we learn from are community health workers (CHWs). Large institutions that are part of our collaborative, including the hospital and the largest social service provider, began building a CHW workforce before the onset of the COVID-19 pandemic, and during the pandemic local CHW positions grew in number and importance. In planning the health department's pandemic response, Ledge Light Health District posted an open CHW position for several months without success. During this time, FRESH New London, a food-justice organization and partner on the Health Improvement Collaborative, hired community member and advocate Lizbeth Polo-Smith to do part-time community engagement work for them. With so much alignment and crossover between the bodies of work of our organizations, it was a natural fit for Ledge Light Health District to also hire Lizbeth as a part-time CHW. Here again was an opportunity for the health department to set bureaucracy and preconceived ideas aside and let the expert do her work. In virtually no time, we saw a much-needed shift in the demographics of people coming to our COVID-19 vaccination clinics; many of those folks continue to engage with us today because of and through Lizbeth.

3. **Talk about power.** If the goal of our community engagement work is to actually dismantle structural racism and to improve the conditions in which our community members "live, work, pray, and play," then we have to be prepared to use our power and privilege to challenge the status quo. This has included topics and conversations both internal and external to the Health Improvement Collaborative.

   One significant way we have addressed power dynamics is in the development of our governance structure and documents. At the beginning of 2020, we had set a goal to establish "bylaws" and have organizations sign "membership agreements." Then . . . COVID. Having to pause this work while our focus was diverted to pandemic response, which required examining and improving our community engagement, resulted in a complete reframing of this goal as well as the development of a document that sets out our values and commitment to dismantling systemic racism and systems of oppression. Our "Purposes and Processes" document, adopted by the Health Improvement Collaborative in February 2022, addresses the collaborative's governance, funding, and decision-making in a way that decentralizes power and assures that the large, more robustly funded and staffed organizations at the table cannot control the agenda or work. The document includes community engagement, resource sharing, and understanding power as three of six key approaches. It includes a process for participatory decision-making—we were careful not to call it voting for a reason—that is based on the "fist to five" model (with a shift away from using a fist, a symbolic gesture for many). We do not charge membership dues or expect anyone to "pay to play," but we do invite well-resourced organizations to contribute funding. We also express a commitment to ensuring alignment between funding opportunities and priorities as expressed by community members and in the CHIP; we won't be chasing every grant dollar that comes along but instead thoughtfully pursuing funding that will allow us to do the work our community members have requested and to stay centered in our values while we do so.

Discussions about power are not limited to the internal dynamics of the Health Improvement Collaborative; part of our community engagement work has been navigating those opportunities to use our power (as individuals or member organizations) to bring the voices of community members to systems and policymakers. So, when our community ambassadors expressed concern with the framing of a "healthy weight" priority put forth by the State Office of Health Strategy, we brought that forward and shared their perceptions that the framing was shaming and rooted in racism and bias. In this situation, we activated our power with another organization that holds power to effect change that was important to our community members. Other situations haven't been so easy to navigate. For example, our collaborative did not publicly support the efforts of a coalition of community groups and members to confront the budgeting practices within a local municipality, as technically the municipality is a member of the collaborative. Talking about power and how and when we can activate it for change is an ongoing conversation (which we elaborate in point 6).

4. **What matters to community members matters the most.** As mentioned earlier, community engagement must extend beyond surveys and focus groups to a true bidirectional flow of information that not only takes but also responds to individuals' stories about how they experience life in our community. If we are talking with community members about their experiences, if our relationships with them are transactional and short term around a specific project (like the CHA), and if we are defining the problem according to what we think we know, then we're not really doing community engagement—we're doing community outreach. Engagement requires us to dig deeper, to actively listen, and to be led by community members. We must create spaces for them to connect with each other and us and to allow us to act with them in their interests.

This approach shows up at the systems or project level in both the development and implementation of the CHIP. In 2016 and again in 2019, quantitative and qualitative data led us to include overdose in the CHIP as a priority issue to be addressed, although the 2016 CHIP framed this topic around "opioid abuse." By engaging with community members—both community organizations doing grassroots work and individuals in our community with lived experience—we learned we need to reframe this issue to be about overdoses related to polysubstance use, to eliminate stigmatizing language like "abuse," and to address the systemic barriers that kept many from accessing services and support. In response to what community members shared with us, we designed New London County Coordinated Access, Resources, Engagement and Support, which centers the work of specialized CHWs, called "navigators," who meet people in parks, grocery stores, libraries, residential hotels, and any other setting imaginable to offer information and support, with whatever the person wants in that moment. Most times, initial engagements are centered around food, transportation, or housing, with no discussions about substance use happening until the navigator has shown that we are worthy of the person's trust because we showed up and responded to what that person, that community member, not we, thought mattered.

5. **Balance the urgency of now with the time it takes.** Mentioned earlier were the delays in filling positions; it wasn't that we had *no* candidates, but that we just didn't have candidates who had the relationship and engagement skills we were hoping for; nor were they bilingual. We could have rushed to fill an open position with one of these candidates and in the past might have. But our work to dismantle structural racism has led us to have different conversations now, and we recognize, as one of our team members commented, "Urgency can serve white supremacy." Had we hired someone who was not bilingual, not connected *to* the community, not *of* the community, we would have been able to check that deliverable off our list, but we would have significantly set back our community engagement work before it even began.

   This idea of resisting urgency is so important when talking about community engagement. We *need* to feel the urgency of health—of lives being negatively affected by systems, policies, and practices—and we need to heed the calls community members have been making for decades (centuries, really) to change things. We cannot pretend time doesn't matter. And yet, it matters so very much. Systems, including the public health system, have continually and repeatedly perpetrated harm, participated in oppression, and let community members down. When we talk about medical mistrust among Black Americans, we must realize that the mistrust is very much earned,

> We have a responsibility to work to earn community members' trust—by showing up, by listening, by following through, by telling the truth when we can't do something, by listening to and sharing their stories with care and intention, and by sharing power and deferring decisions to the community whenever we can.

a protective factor stemming from documented harms like that perpetrated by the Tuskegee Experiment, Henrietta Lacks, Dr. Sims, and so many others, but also resulting from regular lived experiences in doctor's offices, for example, every day, in every community. Resisting urgency thus requires us to be patient.

We must invest the time in building relationships and demonstrate that we will do these things (e.g., listening, caring, and sharing) not just once but repeatedly until doing them becomes the regular way we do things.

6. **Keep on keeping on.** We've shared some pretty phrases here, and it may sound as if we have this community engagement thing down pat, but don't let us fool you—we have so far to go. And we've made so many mistakes and hit so many roadblocks. And we will again—and so will you. Grant funders are not always going to allow flexibility. Project periods are not always going to allow for the time it takes to build relationships. Systems of power are going to continue to be systems of power, and they are going to continue to dictate a lot of what any health department or community collaborative can do. And individuals doing the work, however well intentioned they are, are going to continue to carry the biases and racialized constructs that have been taught to them over and over again. We have failed and you will too. We need to learn to "fail upward," to process what happened and why and move forward with that new information and skills to do better. We must keep on keeping on. Our community members deserve no less.

RHODE ISLAND

Ana P. Novais

The Rhode Island Health Equity Zone (HEZ) mission is to build a healthy and resilient Rhode Island by investing in communities and their capacity to effect change, by honoring the expertise of those who live and work in those communities, and by challenging the systems and structures that perpetuate health inequities.

Rhode Island is the smallest state, geographically, in the entire country, and there are no city or county health departments to serve our one million residents. We sometimes struggle to work at both the macro and micro levels simultaneously. We absolutely rely on partners to be our local voice, to help us carry out community-based programs that help people and the places they call home become healthier.

Over the past decade, Rhode Island has made strides in some areas of public health, as have other states. Tobacco use is down for adults and for youth; also, responsible sexual behavior in adolescents is improving, and teen pregnancy rates are down. However, in other areas, we've had setbacks. Rates of obesity and overweight have gone up, with diabetes and hypertension following the same trend. And more people, particularly people without jobs, are suffering from behavioral health conditions.

Local urban communities in Rhode Island continue to have a higher burden of disease and have had difficulties in coming together to address and improve their health outcomes. Our core cities have the highest concentration of racial and ethnic minority populations, with the lowest social and economic indicators, and our communities struggle for ways to have a more meaningful, sustainable, and impactful engagement with the state.

And for the first time in modern years, the next generation, our children's generation, has a lower life expectancy. One cannot but ask, how can this be? We have all become far too comfortable and complacent with dire statistics and numbers. How can anyone be comfortable with this fact, knowing that it does not have to be this way? Why isn't everyone stopping to consider what is it that we are not doing well? How can we reverse this trend?

At the Rhode Island Department of Health (RIDOH), it became very clear to us that we needed to do public health differently. We needed to change course so that we wouldn't find ourselves a decade from now asking the same questions and seeing further decline in the health of people living in this great state.

We've known for a long time that many forces beyond genetics determine the health of families and children. And so, we factored those determinants into our research and our planning for the next decade and beyond.

It's not just about the how well an individual does, and it's not just about individual choices and individual responsibility; it's about how well our communities "perform," how well our neighborhoods are or how good our school systems and our social supports and services are; it's about the social responsibility of our communities and neighborhoods as a whole—because we know that while genetic makeup offers both protective and risk factors for disease conditions and life trajectories, inequality in health and life outcomes is what has an outsize impact on one's health and well-being.

We knew we needed to change how to do public health, moving away from a medical model that emphasized clinical interventions, counseling, and education (telling people what to do) to focus on addressing the root causes of inequality. We needed to turn all the things we knew into a dynamic strategy that would tackle health problems on all fronts. This led us to take a new approach, adapted from Thomas Frieden's

> We focused on the impact today's experiences and exposures have on tomorrow's health, as well as on the ways key periods in a person's life—infancy, early childhood, and adolescence, for example—are particularly important times for laying the foundations for lifelong physical and mental well-being. And we knew to look at how the elements of the broader social world—education, crime, employment, housing, income—for all affect an individual's and a community's capacity to be healthy.

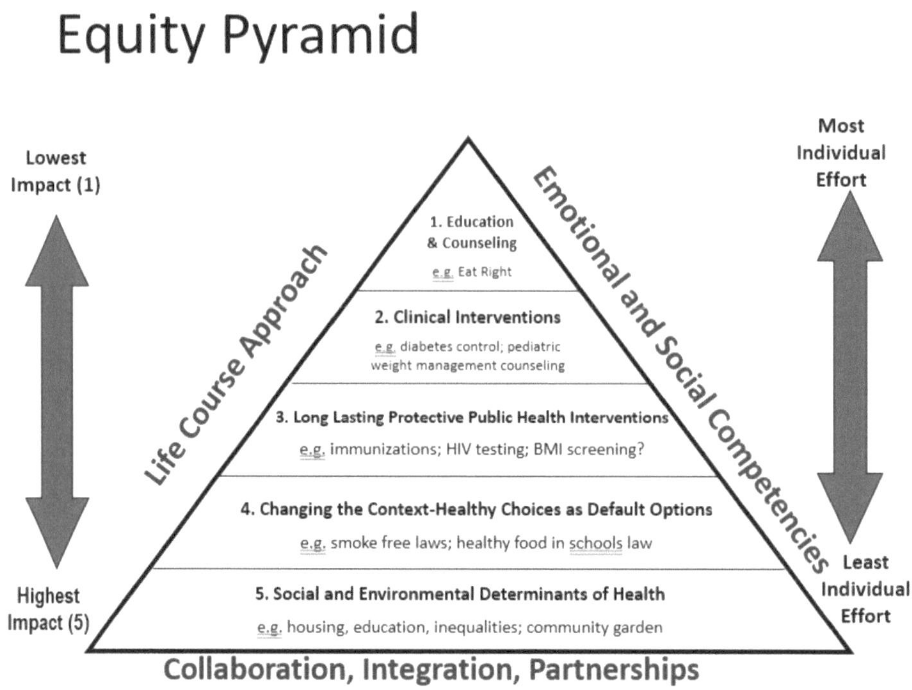

Source: Adapted from Frieden.[5]

Figure 5-2. Rhode Island Health Equity Pyramid: A Framework for Action

"health impact pyramid," which we renamed and presented in *RI Health Equity Pyramid: A Framework for Action* (see Figure 5-2, Rhode Island Health Equity Pyramid: A Framework for Action).[5]

Our first attempt to do public health differently was the Centers for Health Equity and Wellness (CHEW) initiative, which RIDOH established and funded from 2012 to 2015. This project aimed to champion, build capacity for, and sustain community organizations that were already working in the low-income urban neighborhoods in Rhode Island. Each community-based agency or organization applied for funding to address a priority project identified by the local community. The CHEWs each defined their communities in different ways. Some delivered programs to specific population groups, whereas others focused on geographic areas. While we had good intentions, it soon became clear that we weren't giving CHEWs the proper departmental support they required for enduring success. In particular, the initiative did not deliver on the level of power-sharing, community engagement, and self-determination that we had originally promised. As a result, the CHEW communities did not feel sufficiently connected with the projects and programs they were supposed to create.

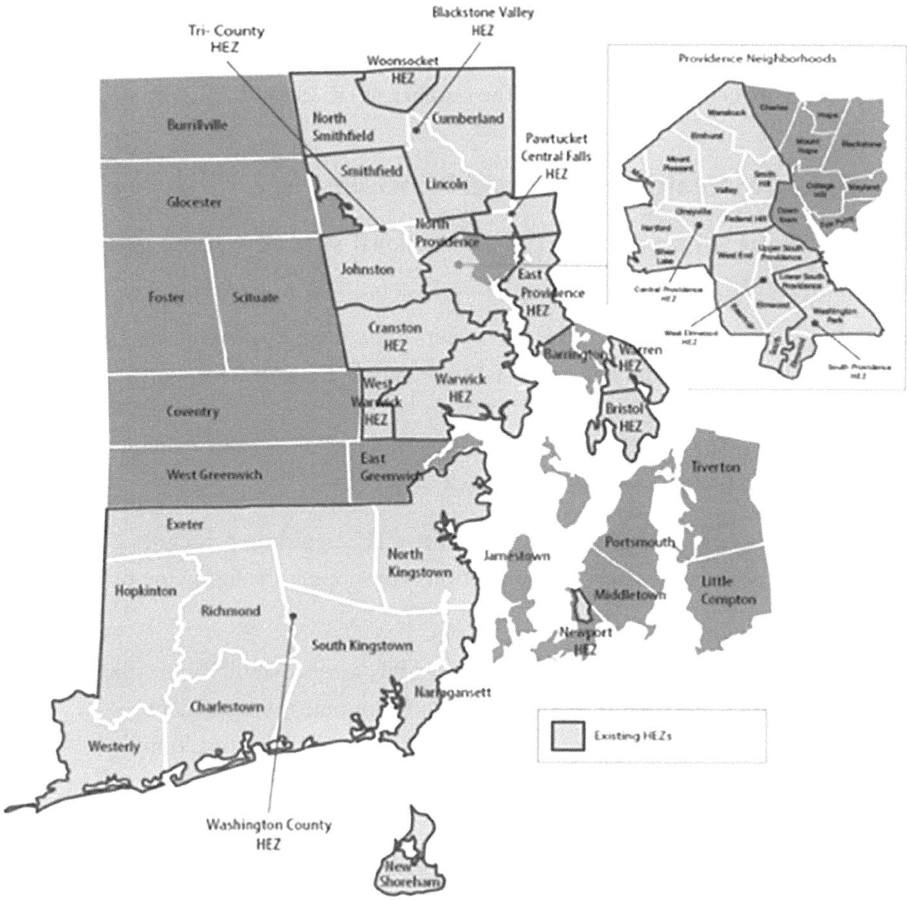

Source: Reprinted with permission from Rhode Island Department of Health.

Figure 5-3. Rhode Island Health Equity Zone Map

The upshot of this shift is that RIDOH is now partnering with community organizations throughout the state to create HEZs. These zones are geographic areas where we harness local engagement to take on the determinants that affect birth outcomes, maternal and child health, and overall population health, all through the lens of equity and collective impact (see Figure 5-3, Rhode Island Health Equity Zone Map).

> So, we shifted gears: we moved from a siloed diseased-focused approach toward a comprehensive community development approach that is place based and that relies on authentic community input and engagement. We took discrete pots of funding we had previously used to target specific diseases, like diabetes, and pooled them to address community issues more broadly—the very ones that perpetuate health inequality.

Rhode Island HEZ's first cohort launched in 2015. We established 10 community partnerships embracing the HEZ theory of change and guiding principles. A second cohort was launched in 2019, bringing the number of HEZs to 15.

Rhode Island Health Equity Zone Principles

The HEZ theory of change is in fact a conditional statement whose parts interact as follows:

If Rhode Island collaboratively invests together* in defined geographic areas to develop sustainable infrastructure and aligns a diverse set of resources to support community-identified needs,

Then positive impacts on the social and environmental conditions driving disparities and poor health outcomes will be demonstrated.

In addition to the HEZ theory of change, five HEZ guiding principles govern our approach as a community-based organization. We support the following process:

1. Define the geographic location for activities.
2. Conduct local assessment of gaps and community assets to establish baseline.
3. Ensure stakeholders' commitment and level of community engagement.
4. Fully engage to develop and implement a community-led plan of action.
5. Put in place a long-term sustainability plan.

The goals for each Rhode Island HEZ community are to improve the population health outcomes and the social and environmental conditions at the neighborhood or place level. This place-based approach calls for collective impact, greater program integration, and values-based decision-making. The public health department developed tools supporting community needs and assets assessment, supported local leadership and staff engagement, and invested in staff and community development. This collaboration brought to life a shared vision of what a healthy community is—one that starts at the local level and is intentionally supported and aligned with a state vision of a healthy state.

A core component of the approach is evidence of the meaningful, true engagement of community stakeholders from the local housing authority, the local education agency, and city hall as well as from community health and mental health centers, community-based organizations, residents, and youth organizations. Shifting the power from state government to a community-led approach means putting the community in the driver's

*Referring to public and private organizations, members of the HEZ collaboratives, as well as state agencies and philanthropic organizations all coming together and agreeing to invest in community identified needs.

seat while the state takes a backseat role and thereby supporting the vision of the community.

Key aspects of any successful framework for a true community-led strategy include relationship building, transparency, clear communication, and effective goal setting, all leading to development and implementation of a plan of action.

Today, Rhode Island has 15 HEZs across the state—15 strong community collaboratives supported by strong-backbone organizations bringing together community stakeholders (organizations and individuals, local government, and school districts), deciding what health means to them, deciding what priorities they want to address, and using evidence-based strategies to implement plans of action that will lead to success.

As with any new initiative, sustainability and scalability are issues that both the department of health and our community partners are engaged in and committed to tackle together. Leadership of the public health department is mindful of the key challenges ahead:

- Funding: the need to create stable funding to sustain the HEZ infrastructure separate from the blended funding approach that the department of health created, as there's no dedicated funding for place-based, equity initiatives;
- Sustainability: how to align with other major health reform initiatives in the state; how to get other decision makers to fully embrace this "health in all policies approach" as the only possible way to truly address the inequalities in health created by poverty; and
- Ownership: local community versus state control.

The power shift at the core of this strategy has been embraced by our HEZ collaboratives, which have pursued additional funding on their own using their community-driven plan of action and priorities. Our HEZs are forging more on-the-ground relationships and launching initiatives that create neighborhood change and foster environments that support healthy choices and healthy living for all residents.

Rhode Island HEZ work plans and activities connect residents to jobs, support small businesses, and address adolescent and behavioral health challenges, chronic diseases, and maternal and child health, in the process taking on everything from transportation to property redevelopment, to financial stability for residents. Rhode Island now has a state health department that has changed the way it does business to partner with communities to address health at the local level through the root causes of inequality and disease. The state has also made a concerted effort to streamline its state-level health policies and programs to further support the implementation of this new strategy and relies on all HEZ stakeholders to push for policies that back this kind of comprehensive approach as the only way to truly address the inequalities in health created by poverty.

At the height of the COVID-19 pandemic, Rhode Island leverage this on-the-ground structure to further support and improve the state's response. The impact of the HEZs

Does achieving health equity seem like a pipe dream? In Rhode Island, we don't think so. We think we can do it, by collaborating with many partners, by listening to residents, by directing resources at the various social determinants of health. We can achieve health equity by bringing social justice to bear on the underlying, social, and environmental roots of disease.

was deeply felt, creating a more targeted response, one that was culturally and linguistically appropriate, bringing testing, vaccine treatment, education, quarantine, and isolation supports to the hard-hit BIPOC communities. The response was, once again, community informed and community led.

This is a matter of life and death—plain and simple. The proposed shift in approach, changing how one does public health, shifting investments to address root causes, building and expanding HEZs across the state and across the US, all of this is in an effort to increase life expectancy and decrease the number of black and brown lives lost to racial inequities. And in our tiny state of Rhode Island, we are racing against big problems, against time, and against the kind of inequality that makes lives harder and cuts them shorter. Getting to good health is a collective project. As a society, we have a responsibility to make sure that all people, no matter where they start out, have access to a good education, a comfortable, safe home, and a pathway to reach their potential. And we need to ensure that everyone has the same chance to live a healthy, productive life. By letting the voice of the community ring strong, Rhode Island is making it happen.

REFERENCES

1. Minkler M. *Community Organizing and Community Building for Health and Welfare.* New Brunswick, NJ: Rutgers University Press; 2012.
2. 10 Essential Public Health Services Futures Initiative Task Force. 10 Essential Public Health Services. September 9, 2020. https://phnci.org/uploads/resource-files/EPHS-English.pdf.
3. Natural Resource Defense Council. Fighting for safe drinking water in Flint. NRDC. April 13, 2022. Accessible at: https://www.nrdc.org/flint. Accessed August 29, 2022.
4. Dissell R, Zeltner B. Toxic neglect: curing Cleveland's legacy of lead poisoning. The Plain Dealer. Updated October 20, 2015. Accessible at: https://www.cleveland.com/healthfit/2015/10/toxic_neglect_curing_cleveland.html. Accessed August 31, 2022.
5. Frieden TA. Framework for public health action: the health impact pyramid. *Am J Public Health.* 2010;100(4):590–595.

Contributors

Lisa Beczkiewicz, Health Promotion Supervisor and Invest Health Team Leader
Missoula City-County Health Department
(missoulacounty.us/government/health/health-department)

Lisa Beczkiewicz has spent the last 20 years in a leadership capacity working to address prevention strategies and health disparities. As Health Promotion Supervisor at the Missoula City-County Health Department, she directs the development, implementation, and evaluation of population health programs in chronic disease, substance use, relationship violence, behavioral health, and injury prevention. She focuses on health equity across all community sectors to provide an opportunity for a person to lead a healthy life. She is data driven and listens to community voices in all her work.

Lisa is the team leader for Missoula Invest Health, a health equity initiative that connects community development and health. With a bachelor's degree in social work from Indiana University and a Certificate in Public Health, she is currently working to complete her master's degree in public health from the University of Montana. Her passion for public health comes from previous work experiences as the supervisor of the Flagship Program, Missoula's largest after-school program; as the executive director of Women in Action, a nonprofit organization working to provide affordable and accessible health and education services in a rural Montana community; and as the coordinator of 5210 Let's Move! Missoula, a childhood obesity prevention collaboration based at the health department.

James Bell III, DSW, Founding Principal
Just Solutions LLC (itsjbthree.my.canva.site)

Dr. James Bell III is Founding Principal of Just Solutions. Just Solutions seeks to equip and empower institutions with the resources and training to reimagine systems through diversity, equity, and inclusion strategies. As a strategic leader, James has demonstrated expertise in driving organizational change within technology and service delivery efforts to drive quality improvement and stakeholder engagement. He has a track record of implementing programs to improve outcomes and establish partnerships with community-based organizations to better serve marginalized and at-risk populations.

James has developed a practice and research trajectory in health disparities and inequities, emphasizing the policy context and health outcomes of African Americans. He has been able to pursue and lead projects to advance equity in both the public and nonprofit sectors. James has been recognized as a thought leader in the areas of health inequities and disparities, social justice, and social innovation. He has presented broadly on these topics, and his passion for this work is evident in his personal, academic, and professional life.

James earned his bachelor's in psychology and master's in social work from Michigan State University. He earned his doctoral degree in social work from the University of Southern California with a focus on the intersection of race, racism, and health. Aside from his professional pursuits, James is also the host of the Equity Matters Podcast, a collection of voices, amplified, sharing in the struggle for social justice and thriving for equity in all sectors.

Natasha Butler, CHW, CHWI, Executive Director
Maternal Upstream Management
(buildhealthchallenge.org/communities/maternal-upstream-management-mum)

As a resident of the Alief community, Natasha Butler has been a community advocate for 20 years. She served as an Alief ISD School Board trustee from 2017 to 2021 and continues to serve as an active member of various organizations, including Alief Super Neighborhood Council, Citgo Innovation Academy at Olle STEM Advisory Board, Community Centered Health Advisory Council, Maternal Upstream Management, Harris County Houston Sports Authority, and March of Dimes Greater Houston Collective Impact. Natasha is an alumna of Harris County Leadership ISD and The BUILD Health Challenge's third cohort. Currently, she serves as a City of Houston Ambassador for Fair Housing and Community Development and Complete Communities Initiative. She is also the founder of Spice Lane Community Investment Group and Westwood Community Investment Group, which promote community development by advocating for access to healthy food, housing, health care, education, and employment through intentional collaboration of local real estate developers, city officials, nonprofits, and residents.

Manuel J. Castañeda, MS, MJ, Director of Community Health
New Brunswick Tomorrow (linkedin.com/in/manuel-j-castaneda-717509b5)

Manuel J. Castañeda serves as Director of Community Health for New Brunswick Tomorrow (NBT). In this role, he manages NBT's Health Task Force and co-facilitates the Healthier New Brunswick network, which takes a comprehensive collective impact approach to improve the overall health of city residents. His work includes strategy building and collaborations with task force volunteers, local stakeholders, and community members in understanding and responding to the health, human services, and educational needs of city residents. He generates ideas and initiatives that affect neighborhoods and aim at engaging the community.

Manuel has extensive client advocacy and case management experience with expertise in health-related legal and benefit/entitlement areas. As the statewide legal services manager for the Hyacinth AIDS Foundation, he managed a statewide legal services program providing legal and client advocacy services for New Jersey residents living with and affected by HIV/AIDS. He also served as editor of the second edition of *AIDS and the Law in New Jersey* (2006). Through his work at the Central Jersey Legal Services Corporation, he provided both assistance and education in areas such as social security disability, Medicaid, benefit/entitlement programs, and immigration. At Rutgers University, he served as a case manager for the Robert Wood Johnson Pediatric AIDS Program, and he continues to serve as an adjunct professor at Rutgers University School of Health Professions. Manuel has a BA and an MS from Rutgers University and an MJ from Loyola University Chicago.

Jodi Cunningham, PhD, Director of Health & Housing
The Community Builders, Inc. (tcbinc.org)

Dr. Jodi Cunningham serves as Community Life Director of Health and Housing at The Community Builders (TCB), a nonprofit affordable housing organization. She supports the Community Life Department by leveraging the platform of TCB's affordable housing to address complex neighborhood health issues through the development of programming, building health partnerships and fund development efforts. Jodi joined TCB in 2017 as a project manager, leading an innovative resident-led health initiative designed to combat infant mortality in the Avondale neighborhood of Cincinnati, Ohio. Drawing on learnings from her health and housing work in Cincinnati, she now works with other staff, partners, and residents to expand TCB's health and housing impact to other communities, including Detroit, Cleveland, Chicago, and Baltimore.

Before joining TCB, Jodi worked in public health, research, academia, and the nonprofit sector, leading efforts ranging from substance abuse prevention to maternal and child health programs. She holds a PhD in health promotion and education, specializing in maternal and child health.

Patrick J. Cusick, MSPH, REHS, Acting Commissioner of Environment
Cleveland Department of Public Health (clevelandhealth.org)

Patrick J. Cusick has been working on improving interdepartmental and interagency efforts in public health for 25 years. His background includes environmental health, emergency preparedness, disease surveillance, and public health epidemiology. He earned his bachelor of arts in biology from Hiram College and a master of science in public health from Walden University. He is a registered environmental health specialist with the State of Ohio.

Patrick has extensive experience working with civic groups, government, and private organizations and other divisions within the city and nationally on environmental issues, emergency preparedness and response, disease surveillance, and operations management in the public and private sector interface. He has been partnering with agencies using those skills to assist in The Build Health Challenge efforts (as awardee in the first and second cohorts and as mentor in the third cohort) to address health equity and access to information, aligning public health, health care, and community advocacy partners to address lead poisoning and asthma prevention, mitigation, and intervention. His work on the City of Cleveland Interdepartmental Healthy Housing Initiative and related efforts were instrumental to restructuring the citywide approach to improving efforts to ensure safe, healthy housing for residents.

Evette De Luca, President
The Social Impact Artists (thesocialimpactartists.com)

Evette De Luca has led within the public sector for 18 years. In 2016, she founded her company, The Social Impact Artists (SIA), and continues to serve as SIA president. The company's mission is to create a world where all people are happier, connected, whole, and powerful. She is also the community engagement leader for the Healthy Ontario Initiative and partners directly with the City of Ontario to lead transformative climate change, community health, and engagement strategies. Her company has also created the Zūm Up! dance and economic mobility initiative and with Kaiser Permanente the Pequeños Pasos de Salud mental health initiative.

Evette also served for four years as Executive Director of Partners for Better Health, where she used her expertise in building and facilitating broad-based partnerships and strategies across multiple cities and communities in San Bernardino and Riverside counties to build health equity. She codesigned and led the Center for Civic Policy & Leadership, an innovations project funded by the California Wellness Foundation that accelerated strategic and collaborative advocacy and policy efforts between government and private and public agencies in the Inland Region. Evette also served as Executive Director of Latino Health Collaborative (LHC), a coalition of more than 40 health-based government and nonprofit organizations that convened the Healthy San Bernardino Coalition. Prior to working for LHC, she served as Executive Director of Foothill Family Shelter, a transitional housing continuum of care with wraparound health, support, and financial services. She holds a master's degree in social impact from Claremont Lincoln University, and she received a bachelor of science in history from UCLA.

Kim Foreman, Executive Director
Environmental Health Watch (ehw.org)

Kim Foreman graduated from Case Western Reserve University in 2001 with a degree in sociology. As Executive Director for Environmental Health Watch in Cleveland, she has focused on environmental justice issues and adverse outcomes of environmental exposures, both indoors and outdoors, that disproportionately affect poor and minority communities.

Kim has developed, implemented, and managed various local and national direct service on the ground, in grassroots projects and has spoken at local and national conventions and appeared on several radio and television shows. She has also been interviewed by the *Cleveland Plain Dealer* and *New York Times* and been featured in the Aljazeera English documentary *Poison in Our Walls.* She has received numerous awards, among them the 2022 National Impactful 40 Enterprise Community Partners Award, 2021 NAACP Unsung Heroes Award, 2019 Cleveland Champions (*Guardian/Cleveland Plain Dealer*), 2019 Ohio Environmental Council Community Collaboration Award, 2019 Ohio State Legislature Environmental Achievement Award, and 2019 Cleveland City Council Resolution of Appreciation.

Sarah Garber, MS, Coordinator for Health Equity
Missoula City-County Health Department

Sarah Garber is Coordinator for Health Equity at Missoula City-County Health Department. She is dedicated to the department's broad-based community-organizing initiative and helps support neighborhood and other equity-based community-organizing efforts. She has also been involved in developing and coordinating stakeholder and partner meetings with local, state, and federal agencies, health care coalitions, other health care partners, and members of the community. She has a passion for building relationships and making Missoula an equitable and inclusive community.

Nichelle Gilbert, Associate Director
Partnership for Community Action (forcommunityaction.org)

Nichelle Gilbert is Associate Director for Partnership for Community Action (PCA). In her role, she manages complex infrastructure and strategic initiatives to build power alongside community toward systems-level change. Nichelle has over 15 years of both lived and professional experience working to support economic and educational success for historically and systematically excluded BIPOC communities. Before working for PCA, Nichelle worked for over a decade in higher education to increase and support a diverse health workforce for New Mexico.

C. Benzel Jimmerson, Founder and Chief Visionary Officer
Metro DEEP, Metropolitan Diversity & Economic Equity Partners (metrodeep.com)

C. Benzel Jimmerson is Founder and CVO of Metro DEEP since 2018, an organization built to align people and partners into ecosystems to improve the well-being and economic mobility of African-descended people in urban settings. He is a serial entrepreneur with equity in eight other companies in the role of strategy development with a goal of building a tribe of 100 companies and the people we love as a part of them. Working since 2000 in direct service related to fatherhood, college admissions, youth engagement, organization leadership, and civic engagement, Benzel has worked with more than 3,000 people. It was this range of experiences that led him to fully commit to economic development as his "lane" and the core issue beyond race that he recognized was of critical importance to the health and future orientation of a community.

Benzel is the father of eight and considers this role to be his most important work. He is also part of the Colorado Black Leadership Coalition, Denver African American Philanthropist, and many other civic-facing organizations. He loves the outdoors, enjoys traveling, and maintains an intimate connection to athletics, which saved his life when he was younger.

Melissa Monbouquette, MPA, Deputy Director
The BUILD Health Challenge (buildhealthchallenge.org)

Melissa Monbouquette is Deputy Director of The BUILD Health Challenge (BUILD), a national initiative that advances multisector, community-driven partnerships to improve health equity. She serves as a thought leader and key resource for awardees and partners by guiding BUILD's strategy and implementation and leads the program's innovation practices to drive sustainable improvements in community health.

Melissa has extensive experience in nonprofit strategy and operation and is dedicated to ensuring communities have what they need to thrive. Before her current role, she served as a program officer with the de Beaumont Foundation, where she managed a portfolio of projects focused on strengthening public health practice through policy development, collaboration, and workforce development. She holds a master's degree from The George Washington University Trachtenberg School of Public Policy and Public Administration and a bachelor's degree from Tufts University.

Jennifer Muggeo, MPH, Deputy Director
Ledge Light Health District (llhd.org)

Jennifer Muggeo is Deputy Director of Ledge Light Health District, located in New London, Connecticut, where she has held a leadership position since March 2007. Throughout her tenure at Ledge Light, she has been fortunate to have the opportunity to merge her skills in business administration with her commitment to supporting community health and addressing inequities. In her roles cochairing both the Health Improvement Collaborative of Southeastern Connecticut and the Overdose Action Team of Southeastern Connecticut, she has emphasized a commitment to supporting people who have been oppressed and placed at risk by systems of care. Her responsibilities include centering Ledge Light Health District's and the Health Improvement Collaborative's commitment to addressing racism as a public health issue and dismantling structural racism and white supremacy.

Jennifer lives in New London with her husband, three children, four guinea pigs, three reptiles, and two pit bulls, all of whom she feels very lucky to come home to each night.

Jessica Mulcahy, MA, Director, Success Measures Philanthropic Evaluation Strategies NeighborWorks America (successmeasures.org)

Jessica Mulcahy is a participatory evaluator and cultural anthropologist who centers equity in her work. By helping individuals and communities define both the issues of challenge and the change they envision, she brings diverse perspectives together for input to evaluative learning and decision-making that respectfully engage community residents. Jessica works in partnership with national funders and intermediaries and their grantees to learn together about the impact of their strategies, investments, and programs in the communities they serve. She also leads the research and development of measurement tools and evaluation frameworks on community development, financial capability, health and healthy communities, affordable housing, and community engagement.

Earlier in her career, Jessica was a research associate at McAuley Institute focusing on the development of the Success Measures evaluation approach and Success Measures Data System. She served as the program coordinator at the Community Partnership Center at University of Tennessee and as the director of the Community Outreach Partnership Center at University of Florida. Jessica holds a bachelor of arts in cultural anthropology from Bryn Mawr College and a master of arts in cultural anthropology from the University of Florida.

Ana P. Novais, Acting Secretary
Rhode Island Executive Office of Health and Human Services

Ana P. Novais currently serves as Acting Secretary for the Rhode Island Executive Office of Health and Human Services. She is deeply involved with Rhode Island's diverse communities and is a board member of various national and state organizations. Ana started at the Rhode Island Department of Health in 1998 as an education and outreach coordinator and, later, as the minority health coordinator, assuring the health needs of the BIPOC communities of Rhode Island were addressed. As the executive director, Ana led the department in the areas of chronic disease, environmental health, and maternal and child health; she focused on developing and implementing the "Rhode Island Health Equity Framework," a plan of action for achieving health equity at the state and local levels through the Health Equity Zones initiative. In 2015, she was promoted to the position of deputy director of health.

Ana earned a clinical psychology degree from UCLN, Belgium, and is a graduate of the Northeastern Public Health Leadership Institute, University of Albany, New York, and Leadership RI. Her career in public health started in 1985 (Cape Verde) and includes five years in Portugal. In the United States, her career has involved her working as a clinical psychologist addressing behavioral health and substance use disorders, as well as providing culturally competent counseling services at local community mental health centers in Rhode Island and Massachusetts.

Ana was born and raised in Cabo Verde, and her roots include Portugal (mother) and Angola (father). Fluent in Creole, Portuguese, French, Spanish, and English, she is a proud mother of four adult children and grandmother to five beautiful youngsters, and loves spending time with family and friends, traveling, reading, photography, and gardening.

Emily Yu, MBA, Executive Director
The BUILD Health Challenge (buildhealthchallenge.org)

As Executive Director of The BUILD Health Challenge (BUILD), Emily Yu is helping to change the future of health in America and leading the charge to cultivate cross-sector collaborations that are working to give everyone a fair chance to be healthy. Skilled in program development and social marketing strategy implementation, for both the public and private sectors, Emily brings together a unique perspective that fuels her passion for both identifying and proving sustainable models for social change.

A dynamic funding collaborative, BUILD is driving sustainable improvements in community health—by improving the social and environmental conditions we less readily associate with health. In support of this bold goal, Emily is forging dynamic partnerships with leading foundations, community-based organizations, hospitals and health systems, public health departments, companies, and others to tackle a wide variety of issues, including improving substandard housing stock, eliminating food deserts, creating opportunities for exercise and active living, and ending the cycle of domestic and gang violence, among others.

Emily earned a master of business administration from New York University's Stern School of Business and a bachelor of science from Georgetown University's Walsh School of Foreign Service. She serves on the Grantmakers in Health Board and was named a 2020 Field Catalyst Fellow with the Center for Community Investment and a 2018 Terrance Keenan Institute for Emerging Leaders in Health Philanthropy Fellow.

Index

Note: Italicized page references indicate Figures, Tables, or Illustrations.

L

M

N

O

P

R

S

T

U

V

W

Y